Preparat
Revision
MRCS and AFRCS

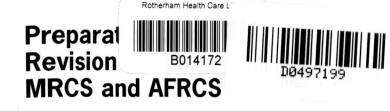

For Churchill Livingstone:

Commissioning editor: Laurence Hunter
Project editor: Barbara Simmons
Copy editor: Colin Nicholls
Project controller: Frances Affleck
Design direction: Erik Bigland

Preparation and Revision for the MRCS and AFRCS

or *How to pass the exam!*

W. E. G. Thomas BSc MBBS FRCS MS

Consultant Surgeon, Royal Hallamshire Hospital, Sheffield;
Court of Examiners, Royal College of Surgeons of England;
Intercollegiate Panel of Examiners;
Surgical Skills Tutor and Hunterian Professor,
Royal College of Surgeons of England;
Moynihan Fellow, Association of Surgeons of Great Britain and Ireland

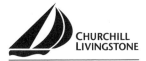

CHURCHILL
LIVINGSTONE

EDINBURGH LONDON NEW YORK PHILADELPHIA SYDNEY TORONTO 1999

CHURCHILL LIVINGSTONE
A Division of Harcourt Brace and Company Limited

Churchill Livingstone, 1–3 Baxter's Place, Leith Walk,
Edinburgh EH1 3AF

Originally published in 1986 as Preparation and Revision for
the FRCS.

ISBN 0443 050465

British Library of Cataloguing in Publication Data
A catalogue record for this book is available from the British
Library.

Library of Congress Cataloging in Publication Data
A catalog record for this book is available from the Library
of Congress.

Medical knowledge is constantly changing. As information
becomes available, changes in treatment, procedures,
equipment and the use of drugs become necessary. The author
and publisher have, as far as it is possible, taken care to
ensure that the information given in the text is accurate and
up-to-date. However, readers are strongly advised to confirm
that the information, especially with regard to drug usage,
complies with current legislation and standard of practice.

Printed in Great Britain by Bell and Bain Ltd., Glasgow

The
publisher's
policy is to use
**paper manufactured
from sustainable forests**

Preface

This book is designed to help candidates in their final preparation for the MRCS and AFRCS examinations. It is not a surgical textbook, nor is it a comprehensive review of the syllabus, but it seeks to help the candidate present his or her knowledge and clinical expertise in a clear, concise and well-formulated manner. The aim is to provide insight as to the nature of the examination by setting out the form for each part, and then to help the candidates in preparing themselves for each section so that they may perform to the very best of their ability.

This is a new examination, and many candidates will be somewhat unsure as to what to expect. Therefore, each section of the examination will be described in detail, including the subject-matter that is examined, and advice given on how best to approach that section. A formal comprehensive revision of the entire syllabus would not be practical, and in any case is virtually provided in the Distance Learning or STEP course published by the Royal College of Surgeons of England. This book simply seeks to help the candidate collate such knowledge and information, and to present his or her knowledge and clinical skills in a way that will result in the most profitable outcome from this new examination.

The nature of this book means that certain subjects are covered in greater depth than others in order to indicate methods of approach and presentation, while some topics are merely referred to *en passant*. It must be stressed, therefore, that the contents do not represent a complete or exhaustive coverage of the syllabus, but hopefully will stimulate the candidate to further reading as recommended in Appendix 3. Furthermore, this book is not an alternative to such reading, but should be used as an adjunct to it, preferably after appropriate clinical experience and training. Much of the advice given may appear obvious or unnecessary, but, having observed examination candidates at work for several years, I feel that this advice is not only pertinent but needs to be repeated and stressed once more.

Many of the points raised in this book are equally relevant to all clinicians involved in the art and practice of surgery, and it is hoped that its usefulness will not be restricted to candidates sitting the MRCS or AFRCS examinations. Inevitably such a volume reflects, to a degree, a personal view of many of the topics covered, and it is not intended to suggest that the advice given is the only profitable method of approach. However, the hints and tips given regarding the multiple-choice papers, the clinical examination and the vivas will, I trust, prove beneficial and help many 'budding' surgeons forward their careers.

Acknowledgements
I wish to acknowledge gratefully the help and support of many of my clinical colleagues for their critique and encouragement in the preparation of this book. I particularly wish to thank Messrs Gary James and Pat Elliot for much of the artwork, and to the Medical Illustration Departments of the Bristol Royal Infirmary, Royal Devon and Exeter Hospital and the Royal Hallamshire Hospital in Sheffield for their assistance in the preparation of the illustrations. I am most grateful to Ewan Pullen and Sarah Robinson of the Examinations Department of the Royal College of Surgeons of England for their permission to reproduce much of the 'Advice to Candidates' that accompanies the multiple-choice question papers. I also wish to thank my fellow examiners for their 'unbounded wisdom' and my wife for her 'unbounded patience'. Finally I would like to thank all prospective candidates, for without their involvement this book would be totally irrelevant.

Sheffield 1999   W. E. G. Thomas

Contents

The requirements of the examination

1

An introduction to basic surgical training

Basic surgical training (BST) aims to provide a firm surgical and clinical foundation in the general principles of surgery that will equip a trainee surgeon to enter higher surgical training in one of the surgical specialties. It comprises a minimum of 2 years of clinical practice in approved training posts within rotations that provide the mandatory clinical training and adequate opportunities for education rather than routine service commitments alone. It is a totipotential period in which the trainee should participate in audit and be introduced to the practice and principles of research and medical ethics. Trainees should also acquire an adequate knowledge of the basic sciences relevant to surgery and, although the formal and specific examination of them as in the former Primary or Part 1 is no longer conducted, knowledge of clinically related anatomy, physiology and pathology will be assessed in the MCQ papers and in the viva voce examinations. Many trainees will acquire their knowledge of the basic sciences through private study or course attendance, while others may still take posts as demonstrators in university departments, although wherever possible these should be linked to formal basic surgical training programmes (these cannot form part of the minimum 2-year period of clinical training).

Eligibility for the Diploma of MRCS or AFRCS

To be eligible to be awarded the Diploma of MRCS or AFRCS, all candidates must not only have passed all sections of the appropriate examinations but also:

● Possess a primary medical qualification that is acceptable to the United Kingdom General Medical Council for *full registration* or for *limited registration*

- Have satisfactorily completed the prescribed 2-year period of mandatory clinical training (see below)
- Have satisfactorily completed the mandatory Basic Surgical Skills course and received the appropriate certificate and number (see p. 8)
- Hold an authenticated log book of their training (see p. 7)
- Have been engaged in acquiring professional knowledge and training for at least 36 months since obtaining the primary qualification required above
- Have complied with all the regulations and signed a declaration of compliance with all the ordinances of the appropriate college.

Mandatory clinical training

Training programmes

A minimum of 2 years of clinical training is mandatory and this should comprise:

- 6 months in general surgery, or one of its subspecialties, with *general emergency work*
- 6 months in orthopaedics, or one of its subspecialties, with *general musculoskeletal trauma*
- 12 months* either in two other surgical specialties (each of 6 months' duration) or in three other surgical specialties (each of 4 months' duration), as listed below:
  — Accident and Emergency (strongly recommended)
  — cardiothoracic surgery
  — gynaecology
  — neurosurgery
  — ophthalmology
  — oral and maxillofacial surgery
  — otolaryngology
  — paediatric surgery
  — plastic surgery
  — urology
  — pure subspecialties of general surgery or orthopaedics, provided such subspecialty experience has not already been acquired in the mandatory general surgery or orthopaedic posts.

---

* Maxillofacial trainees (with a full or temporary registered dental qualification with the UK General Dental Council) must complete 12 months of oral and maxillofacial surgical training in a post approved by the Faculty of Dental Surgery.

3 months of experience in intensive care will be acceptable as part of the 2-year period of mandatory training. This may be acquired as part of an approved surgical post or as part of a Royal College of Anaesthetists approved 4-month post in anaesthesia with intensive therapy.

All trainees must present evidence of satisfactory completion of this training, which should comprise an authenticated certificate from the local surgical tutor or, if this is not possible, a statement signed by all the trainee's consultant trainers.

Timetable

Every surgical trainee should be part of an identified surgical team and be directly responsible to one or more consultant surgeons who supervise his or her training. Trainees should have a clearly defined role within the clinical team and there must be a balance between training and service commitments. Their timetable should include:

- The diagnosis and treatment of elective and emergency admissions
- Outpatient clinics
- Assisting at operations (performing procedures as and when appropriate)
- Intensive and postoperative care.

Routine service tasks, such as phlebotomy, should only form a very limited part of the workload. In order to assist in the balance of training and service commitments, the following model timetable has been suggested, but should be interpreted flexibly:

Operating (2–3 sessions)
All operations should be recorded in the log book, and operations recorded should differentiate between emergency and elective procedures and as to whether they were performed with or without assistance. Unsupervised procedures should only be undertaken after adequate and appropriate experience with skilled assistance close at hand.

Outpatients (2 sessions)
Trainees should see both new and follow-up patients under the supervision of, and in consultation with, a consultant or higher surgical trainee.

Wardwork (2–3 sessions)
There should be a daily business-round to implement senior surgical staff's instructions, with at least one formal round with the consultant

trainer for teaching purposes. Routine clerking of patients should not trespass on the time in outpatients or in the operating theatre, and trainees should ideally be supported by pre-registration HOs in these duties.

Administration *(1 session)*
Discharge summaries and coding data for audit are an essential part of training and require appropriate secretarial and computer back-up.

Personal study *(1 session)*
Protected time must be set aside during the working week for personal study.

Teaching *(1 session)*
Each BST programme must have a regular schedule of teaching sessions that should include postgraduate meetings, audit, ward-rounds, and departmental and interdepartmental meetings. Experience at presenting cases at such meetings is an essential part of surgical education and opportunities should be afforded regularly.

Emergency and on-call duties
Emergency and on-call duties are an essential part of surgical training, and it is suggested that 32 hours per week of such work is appropriate within a 72-hour working week. Over a 4-week period this allows a 1 in 4 rota to be worked, but this may need to be varied according to the availability of junior staff; if there is the necessity to provide prospective cover for absent colleagues, a 1 in 5 rota is more appropriate. Such emergency work must always be supervised by a consultant or higher surgical trainee in the appropriate specialty.

Skills

Every basic surgical trainee should be given the opportunity to acquire the *general* and the *specialty* clinical and practical skills necessary. A comprehensive list of such skills cannot be provided in this context but the following are listed for guidance:

General skills
- Communication skills with patients, relatives, nursing staff, paramedics, general practitioners, other hospital departments (e.g. X-ray, laboratories)
- Maintenance of clinical and operating notes

- Supervision and support of pre-registration house officers and medical students
- Understanding the role of other departments in diagnosis such as X-ray, ultrasound, CT, radionuclides, endoscopy, biopsy, histopathology, cytology, etc.
- The ability to elicit the symptoms and signs in patients with surgical disorders
- Preoperative assessment of patients (e.g. cardiac, respiratory, renal status, diabetes, hypertension, malnutrition). The selection of patients for operative procedures
- Perioperative management — antibiotics, prevention of DVT and pulmonary embolism
- Postoperative care — indications for intensive care, pain relief, use of antibiotics, care of venous lines and catheters, fluid and electrolyte balance, blood gas analysis, management of common surgical complications, multiple organ failure, terminal care
- Follow-up — need for surveillance in appropriate patients
- Practical skills in safe operating theatre practice (sterility and sterilization), incisions, tissue handling, diathermy (use and safety), wound closure (sutures, needles, knotting technique, staples), simple skin grafting, drains and catheters, life-saving manoeuvres (endotracheal intubation, cardiac massage, chest drain).

Specialty skills

Each specialty offers the opportunity to learn new skills and operative procedures appropriate to basic surgical training. All such procedures should be noted in the log book. It is not appropriate to list all such specialty skills here, but the two main mandatory specialties of general surgery and orthopaedics are listed for illustration purposes.

General surgery

Clinical skills
- Diagnosis and management of acute abdominal emergencies
- Total parenteral nutrition
- Initial assessment and resuscitation of head, chest and abdominal injuries.

Practical skills
- Endoscopy and laparoscopy
- Thoracic and peritoneal aspiration and drainage
- Draining abscesses
- Standard surgical approaches
- Laparotomy

- Removal of simple cutaneous and subcutaneous swellings
- Appendicectomy
- Strangulated hernia
- Bowel resection and anastomosis
- Hernioplasty
- Varicose veins
- Sigmoidoscopy and minor anal-rectal procedures
- Excision of breast lumps.

Orthopaedic surgery

Clinical skills

- Fracture and elective outpatient clinics
- Assessment and management of acute musculoskeletal trauma.

Practical skills

- Aspiration of joints and injection of steroids
- Surgical approach to major bones and joints
- Manipulative reduction of fractures
- Application of splints and plaster casts
- Skeletal traction and external fixation
- Internal fixation of common fractures, including the hip
- Hemi-arthroplasty of the hip joint
- Fusion of small joints of the toes
- Carpal tunnel decompression
- Excision of ganglia
- Common amputations
- Management of injuries to, and infections of, the hand.

Educational facilities

All basic surgical training posts should provide the trainee with the following educational facilities:

Books

There must be a well-supervised library with facilities for evening reading and a borrowing service. Appropriate books should also be available in the Department of Surgery and in the operating theatre.

Study leave

Paid study leave must be available in addition to the weekly sessions for personal study, according to a trainee's entitlement. Leave should be granted for attendance at the mandatory Basic Surgical Skills course (see p. 8) and for other highly recommended courses such as the Advanced Trauma Life Support course (ATLS), as is appropriate.

Living accommodation
There must be suitable living-in accommodation for on-call purposes and adequate food available at all hours.

Facilities for audit
Secretarial services and computer facilities for discharge summaries, data collection and audit must be provided.

Teaching programme
Each BST programme should have regular sessions for postgraduate teaching with departmental and interdepartmental meetings, seminars, audit sessions and tutorials. All trainees should be registered with a postgraduate education programme and hours of attendance recorded. Trainees should also be encouraged to take part in teaching medical students, nurses and paramedical personnel.

Log books
All trainees must maintain a log book throughout their mandatory period of training in which to record their clinical, surgical and educational experience. The log book should contain details of each post undertaken, along with dates, as well as the clinical and operative experience gained during that period. Each operation logged should also provide information as to whether the trainee assisted at, was assisted during, or actually performed unsupervised, each procedure. Furthermore, it should be noted whether the procedure was an elective or emergency one, and whether there were any complications or death resulting. The contents of the log book must be authenticated at regular intervals by the trainee's consultant and his or her overall training supervisor or surgical tutor.

The log book should also contain details of any educational courses attended, along with the dates, as well as the details of the mandatory Basic Surgical Skills course attended, with the certificate of completion and the trainee's personalized certificated number. Approved log books are available from the respective colleges.

Counselling

Surgical tutor
The College surgical tutor and the regional postgraduate dean are both available for career advice and guidance. The regional BST Committee is responsible for monitoring the progress of each trainee, and it is recommended that the trainee be interviewed at regular intervals and a confidential report prepared for discussion with, and countersigning

by, the trainee. Comments by the trainee regarding the training received should be sent to the surgical tutor so that action may be taken to remedy any deficiency.

Appeals

If a trainee considers that:

- He or she has been treated unfairly
- The clinical experience has not met expectations
- Routine service work has been disproportionate to the educational value
- A confidential report seems to be unfair,

then he should talk to the surgical tutor and the hospital clinical tutor. If the outcome of such discussion is not deemed satisfactory, the trainee has the right to seek help from the following successively:

- The College regional adviser and the regional postgraduate dean
- The chairman of the College Training Board
- The president of the appropriate Royal College of Surgeons.

Basic surgical skills — a mandatory training course

All trainees must satisfactorily complete the Intercollegiate Basic Surgical Skills course. This is a 3-day course that consists of three modules:

1. Open surgery ($1\frac{1}{2}$ days)
2. Orthopaedics and trauma ($\frac{1}{2}$ day)
3. Minimal access surgery (1 day).

It is a highly practical course with 'hands-on' experience and a high tutor-to-participant ratio. The presentation is uniform throughout the UK and overseas, and the standard is maintained by means of regular assessments by all the UK surgical colleges and the Irish Surgical College. The content is also standardized by means of the course materials, which include the course video and both participant and faculty handbooks. Each exercise in the course is demonstrated by means of the course video, and then the participants perform that exercise under the guidance and tutorship of the faculty members. At the end of each module there is an assessment exercise which is appraised by the appropriate faculty member. At the end of the course all participants who have satisfactorily completed all the modules will receive a signed certificate containing their own specific number which is maintained on a database at the appropriate college, and the number should be entered into the log book. This inter-collegiate course is recognized by all four colleges, regardless of where it is actually undertaken.

Trainees are also advised to attend other educational courses such as the Advanced Trauma Life Support course (ATLS), which is highly recommended but not mandatory. Other courses as and when developed, such as the Critical Care courses, are also recommended.

Summary

In summary, eligibility for the award of the diploma of MRCS or AFRCS requires that all candidates should:

- Possess a primary medical qualification recognized by the GMC
- Have completed the prescribed 2-year period of mandatory clinical training
- Hold an authenticated log book of their training
- Have satisfactorily completed the mandatory Basic Surgical Skills course
- Have been engaged in acquiring professional knowledge and training for at least 36 months since obtaining their primary qualification
- Have passed all the sections of the MRCS or AFRCS examinations (see Ch. 3)
- Have complied with all the regulations and paid the Diploma Completion Fee
- Have signed, in the presence of an officer of the College, a declaration of compliance with the ordinances of the College.

The syllabus for the examination

2

Introduction

No syllabus for any examination can be comprehensive. However, the UK Surgical Royal Colleges and the Irish Surgical College have reached an agreement as to the basic content and nature of the syllabus for basic surgical trainees and candidates for the MRCS and AFRCS examinations. This agreement is published in two documents entitled *Outline Proposals for the Reform of Basic Surgical Training and Examinations* (July 1995) and *Integrated Syllabus for Basic Surgical Training* (May 1995). These documents describe the content of the syllabus and the means by which it should be delivered. This means that there is now a common syllabus for basic surgical training in which the basic sciences are integrated with clinical surgery in general. The examinations of all four colleges will be based upon such a syllabus and, although each college may alter the presentation of the syllabus to suit its own courses and examinations, the content cannot be changed. Furthermore, the colleges are encouraging the provision of education for basic surgical trainees based on the delivery of this syllabus by means of distance learning and short courses in basic surgical skills and basic patient management skills.

Although the old-style Primary or Part 1 examination no longer exists, candidates are still expected to have a working knowledge of anatomy, physiology and pathology that will enable them to understand the effects of common surgical diseases and injuries upon the normal structure and function of the systems of the human body. They must understand the principles and practice of care of the patient pre-, peri- and postoperatively, including the actions and potential toxicity of drugs used in these situations. They must have a working knowledge of the care of the critically ill patient including the principles of intensive care management. They must have an understanding of trauma management, neoplasia, general pathology including immunology and microbiology, and the techniques and outcome of surgery, as well as such principles as medical ethics and medicolegal issues. They should also have a clinically based working knowledge of the disease processes and clinical conditions affecting the major systems of the body, including:

- The locomotor system
- The vascular system
- The head and neck, endocrine systems and paediatric conditions
- The abdomen
- The urinary system and renal transplantation.

Outline of syllabus

The content of the syllabus can roughly be divided into two basic groupings:

- Principles of Surgery in General
- Systematic Surgery.

The two multiple-choice question papers tend to be based on this division of topics and, indeed, the Royal College of Surgeons of England has based the distance learning course upon it. The Principles of Surgery in General are covered by five core modules entitled:

1. Peri-operative management 1
2. Peri-operative management 2
3. Trauma
4. Intensive care
5. Neoplasia. Techniques and outcome of surgery

The Systematic Surgery is covered by five further system modules that correspond to the systems described above, namely:

A. Locomotor system
B. Vascular
C. Head, neck, endocrine and paediatric
D. Abdomen
E. Urinary system and renal transplantation

For convenience, therefore, the common syllabus, as outlined in the document *Integrated Syllabus for Basic Surgical Training*, has been presented in modular form and is described below. It must be stressed that this syllabus is indicative of the areas of knowledge expected of candidates. It is not intended to be exhaustive or to exclude other items of knowledge which are of similar relevance.

Core module 1: Peri-operative management 1

Pre-operative management

- Assessment of fitness for anaesthesia and surgery
- Tests of respiratory, cardiac and renal function
- Management of associated medical conditions (e.g. diabetes; respiratory disease; cardiovascular disease; psychiatric disorders; malnutrition; anaemia; steroid, anticoagulant, immunosuppressant and other drug therapy).

Infection

- Pathophysiology of the body's response to infection
- The sources of surgical infection — prevention and control
- Surgically important micro-organisms
- Principles of asepsis and antisepsis
- Surgical sepsis and its prevention
- Aseptic techniques
- Skin preparation
- Antibiotic prophylaxis
- Sterilization.

Investigative and operative procedures

- Excision of cysts and benign tumours of skin and subcutaneous tissue
- Principles of techniques of biopsy
- Suture and ligature materials
- Drainage of superficial abscesses
- Basic principles of anastomosis.

Anaesthesia

- Principles of anaesthesia
- Pre-medication
- Local and regional anaesthesia
- Care and monitoring of the anaesthetized patient.

Theatre problems

- Surgical technique and technology
- Diathermy. Principles and precautions

- Lasers. Principles and precautions
- Explosion hazards relating to general anaesthesia and endoscopic surgery
- Tourniquets. Uses and precautions
- Prevention of nerve and other injuries in the anaesthetized patient
- Surgery in hepatitis and HIV carriers (special precautions)
- Disorders of coagulation and haemostasis (prophylaxis of thromboembolic disease).

Core module 2: Peri-operative management 2

Skin and wounds

- Pathophysiology of wound healing
- Classification of surgical wounds
- Principles of wound management
- Incisions and their closure
- Suture and ligature materials
- Wound dehiscence
- Dressings.

Fluid balance

- Assessment and maintenance of fluid and electrolyte balance
- Techniques of venous access
- Nutritional support. Indications, techniques, total parenteral nutrition.

Blood

- Disorders of coagulation and haemostasis
- Blood transfusion. Indications, hazards, complications, plasma substitutes
- Haemolytic disorders of surgical importance
- Haemorrhagic disorders; disorders of coagulation.

Postoperative complications

- Postoperative complications — prevention, monitoring recognition, management
- Ventilatory support — indications.

Postoperative sequelae

- Pain control
- Immune response to trauma, infections and tissue transplantation
- Pathophysiology of the body's response to trauma
- Surgery in the immunocompromised patient.

Core module 3: Trauma

Initial assessment and resuscitation after trauma

- Clinical assessment of the injured patient
- Maintenance of airway and ventilation
- Haemorrhage and shock.

Chest, abdomen and pelvis

- Cardiorespiratory physiology as applies to trauma
- Penetrating chest injuries and pneumothorax
- Rib fractures and flail chest
- Abdominal and pelvic injuries.

Central nervous system trauma

- Central nervous system: anatomy and physiology relevant to clinical examination of the central nervous system; the understanding of its functional disorders, particularly those caused by cranial or spinal trauma; and the interpretation of special investigations
- Intracranial haemorrhage
- Head injuries — general principles of management
- Surgical aspects of meningitis
- Spinal cord injury and compression
- Paraplegia and quadriplegia — principles of management.

Special problems

- Pre-hospital care
- Triage
- Trauma scoring systems
- Traumatic wounds — principles of management

- Gunshot and blast wounds
- Skin loss — grafts and flaps
- Burns
- Facial and orbital injuries.

Principles of limb injury

- Peripheral nervous system: anatomy and physiology
- Fractures — pathophysiology of fracture healing
- Non-union, delayed union, complications
- Principles of bone grafting
- Traumatic oedema, compartment and crush syndrome, fat embolism
- Brachial plexus injury.

Core module 4: Intensive care

Cardiovascular

- The surgical anatomy and applied physiology of the heart relevant to clinical cases
- Physiology and pharmacological control of: cardiac output, blood flow, blood pressure, coronary circulation
- Cardiac arrest, resuscitation
- Monitoring of cardiac function in the critically ill patient, coma, central venous pressure, pulmonary wedge pressure, tamponade, cardiac output measurements
- The interpretation of special investigations
- The management of haemorrhage and shock
- Pulmonary oedema
- Cardiopulmonary bypass; general principles, cardiac support.

Respiratory

- The surgical anatomy of the airways, chest wall, diaphragm and thoracic viscera
- The mechanics and control of respiration
- The interpretation of special investigations; lung function tests, arterial blood gases, radiology
- The understanding of disorders of respiratory function caused by trauma, acute surgical illness and surgical intervention
- Respiratory failure

- Adult respiratory distress syndrome
- Endotracheal intubation, laryngotomy, tracheostomy
- Artificial ventilation.

Multisystem failure

- Multisystem failure
- Renal failure: diagnosis of renal failure, complications of renal failure
- GI tract, hepatic failure
- Nutrition.

Problems in intensive care

- Sepsis, predisposing factors, organisms causing septicaemia
- Complications of thoracic operations
- Localized sepsis, pneumonia, lung abscess, bronchiectasis, empyema, mediastinitis.

Principles of ICU

- Indications for admission
- Organization and staffing
- Scoring
- Costs.

Core module 5: Neoplasia. Techniques and outcome of surgery

Principles of oncology

- Epidemiology of common neoplasms and tumour-like conditions; role of cancer registries
- Clinicopathological staging of cancer
- Pathology; clinical features, diagnosis and principles of management of common cancers in each of the surgical specialties
- Principles of cancer treatment by surgery; radiotherapy; chemotherapy; immunotherapy and hormone therapy
- The principles of carcinogenesis and the pathogenesis of cancer relevant to the clinical features, special investigations, staging and the principles of treatment of the common cancers
- Principles of molecular biology of cancer, carcinogenesis; genetic factors; mechanisms of metastasis.

Cancer screening and treatment

- The surgical anatomy and applied physiology of the breast relevant to clinical examination, the interpretation of special investigations, the understanding of disordered function and the principles of the surgical treatment of common disorders of the breast
- The breast — acute infections; benign breast disorders; nipple discharge; mastalgia
- Carcinoma of the breast; mammography; investigation and treatment
- Screening programmes.

Techniques of management

- Terminal care of cancer patients; pain relief
- Rehabilitation
- Psychological effects of surgery and bereavement.

Ethics and the law

- Medical/legal ethics and medicolegal aspects of surgery
- Communication with patients, relatives and colleagues.

Outcome of surgery

- The evaluation of surgery and general topics
- Decision-making in surgery
- Clinical audit
- Statistics and computing in surgery
- Principles of research and design and analysis of clinical trials
- Critical evaluation of innovations — technical and pharmaceutical
- Health service management and economic aspects of surgical care.

System module A: Locomotor system

Musculoskeletal anatomy and physiology relevant to clinical examination of the locomotor system and to the understanding of disordered locomotor function, with emphasis on the effects of acute musculoskeletal trauma.

Effects of trauma and lower limb

- Effects of acute musculoskeletal trauma
- Common fractures and joint injuries
- Degenerative and rheumatoid arthritis (including principles of joint replacement)
- Common disorders of the foot
- Amputations.

Infections and upper limb

- Common soft tissue injuries and disorders
- Infections of bones and joints (including implants and protheses)
- Pain in the neck, shoulder and arm
- Common disorders of the hand, including hand injuries and infections.

Bone disease and spine

- Common disorders of infancy and childhood
- Low back pain and sciatica
- Metabolic bone disease (osteoporosis, osteomalacia)
- Surgical aspects of paralytic disorders and nerve injuries.

System module B: Vascular

The surgical anatomy and applied physiology of blood vessels relevant to clinical examination, the interpretation of special investigations and the understanding of the role of surgery in the management of cardiovascular disease.

Arterial diseases

- Chronic obliterative arterial disease
- Amputations
- Carotid disease
- Aneurysms
- Special techniques used in the investigation of vascular disease
- Limb ischaemia — acute and chronic; clinical features; gangrene; amputations for vascular disease
- Principles of reconstructive arterial surgery.

Venous diseases

- Vascular trauma and peripheral veins
- Varicose veins
- Venous hypertension, post-phlebitic leg, venous ulceration
- Disorders of the veins in the lower limb
- Deep venous thrombosis and its complications
- Chronic ulceration of the leg
- Thrombosis and embolism.

Lymphatics and spleen

- Thromboembolic disease
- Spleen; splenectomy; hypersplenism
- Lymph nodes; lymphoedema
- Surgical aspects of autoimmune disease
- The anatomy and physiology of the haemopoietic and lymphoreticular systems
- Surgical aspects of disordered haemopoiesis.

System module C: Head, neck, endocrine and paediatric

The surgical anatomy and applied physiology of the head and neck relevant to clinical examination, the interpretation of special investigations, the understanding of disorders of function, and the treatment of disease and injury involving the head and neck.

The head

- Laryngeal disease, maintenance of airway; tracheostomy
- Acute and chronic inflammatory disorders of the ear, nose, sinuses and throat
- Intracranial complications
- Foreign bodies in ear, nose and throat
- Epistaxis
- Salivary gland disease
- The eye — trauma, common infections.

Neck and endocrine glands

The surgical anatomy and applied physiology of the endocrine glands relevant to clinical examination, the interpretation of special investigations, the understanding of disordered function and the principles of the surgical treatment of common disorders of the endocrine glands.

- Common neck swellings
- Thyroid. Role of surgery in diseases of the thyroid; complications of thyroidectomy; the solitary thyroid nodule
- Parathyroid; hyperparathyroidism; hypercalcaemia
- Secondary hypertension.

Paediatric disorders

- Neonatal physiology; the special problems of anaesthesia and surgery in the newborn; the principles of neonatal fluid and electrolyte balance
- Correctable congenital abnormalities
- Common paediatric surgical disorders — cleft lip and palate; pyloric stenosis; intussusception; hernia; maldescent of testis; torsion; diseases of the foreskin.

System module D: Abdomen

The surgical anatomy of the abdomen and its viscera and the applied physiology of the alimentary system relevant to clinical examination, the interpretation of common special investigations, the understanding of disorders of function, and the treatment of abdominal disease and injury.

Abdominal wall

- Anatomy of the groin, groin hernias, acute and elective. Clinical features of hernias, complications of hernias
- Anterior abdominal wall, anatomy, incisions, laparoscopic access.

Acute abdominal conditions

- Peritonitis; intra-abdominal abscesses
- Common acute abdominal emergencies
- Intestinal obstruction; paralytic ileus
- Intestinal fistulae
- Investigation of abdominal pain
- Investigation of abdominal masses
- Gynaecological causes of acute abdominal pain
- Pelvic inflammatory disease
- Abdominal injury.

Elective abdominal conditions

- Common anal and perianal disorders
- Jaundice — differential diagnosis and management
- Portal hypertension
- Gallstones
- Gastrostomy, ileostomy, colostomy and other stomata.

System module E: Urinary system and renal transplantation

The surgical anatomy and applied physiology of the genitourinary system relevant to clinical examination, special investigations, understanding of disordered function, and the principles of the surgical treatment of genitourinary disease and injury.

Urinary tract I

- Urinary tract infection
- Haematuria
- Trauma to the urinary tract
- Urinary calculi.

Urinary tract II

- Retention of urine
- Disorders of the prostate
- Pain and swelling in the scrotum; torsion.

Renal failure and transplantation

- Principles of transplantation
- Renal failure; dialysis.

The format of the examination

3

Introduction

The exact format of the examination will depend upon which Royal College of Surgeons is conducting the proceedings. The detailed description given here is based on the MRCS examination as it is currently conducted by the Royal College of Surgeons of England. However, the examinations for the other colleges are very similar and only vary in detail, and all are based on the identical syllabus with the same standard of knowledge being required. Standards are maintained by having exchange examiners for each college, which ensures that expectations are similar and that the examinations are equivalent. Information as to details of each examination and their timing may be obtained from the appropriate registrars or examination departments for each college (see Appendix 5).

The examination

The Royal College of Surgeons of England

The MRCS Diploma examination consists of:

- The multiple-choice question section
- The clinical section
- The viva voce section.

The multiple-choice question (MCQ) section
- The MCQ section consists of two papers each of 2 hours' duration. The first will be based upon the core modules of the syllabus (see Ch. 2) and the second on the system modules
- Candidates may enter one or both papers on any occasion
- Each paper will stand alone, candidates being awarded either a 'pass' or 'fail'

- Candidates may resit each of the MCQ papers as often as they wish
- There is full reciprocity of recognition of a 'pass' in the MCQ section between all three UK surgical colleges and the Irish Surgical College
- Details as to the make-up of the MCQ papers are given in Chapter 5.

The clinical section

- Candidates must have been awarded a 'pass' in both MCQ papers before entering the clinical section
- Candidates must have completed 20 months of their mandatory clinical training period before entering the clinical section
- The clinical section will last approximately 50 minutes and be based upon five bays of 'short cases' derived from all surgical specialties and be relevant to the whole syllabus. It is likely that these bays will comprise:
  — superficial lesions (lumps and bumps)
  — musculoskeletal and neurological cases (orthopaedics)
  — circulatory and lymphatic cases (vascular)
  — the abdomen and trunk
  — communication skills
  Further details as to the clinical section are given in Chapters 6–11
- Candidates will be awarded a 'pass' or 'fail'
- Candidates will be allowed to take the clinical section examination within the time constraints described below under 'Limits on the Number of Attempts'.

The viva voce section

- Candidates must have been awarded a 'pass' in both MCQ papers and in the clinical section and completed the approved Intercollegiate Basic Surgical Skills course before entering the viva voce section
- Candidates must have completed 22 months of their mandatory clinical training before entering the viva voce section
- The questions in the viva voce section will cover the whole syllabus
- The viva voce section will consist of three vivas lasting 1 hour in total and will comprise:
  — applied surgical anatomy with operative surgery
  — applied physiology and critical care
  — clinical pathology with principles of surgery
  Each viva will last 20 minutes and consist of two 10-minute oral examinations
- Each viva will be conducted by a pair of examiners, except for the Operative Surgery viva, where there will be three examiners to allow the log book to be examined

- Log books *must* be brought to the viva voce section of the examination
- Candidates will be awarded a 'pass' or 'fail'
- Candidates will be allowed to take the viva voce section within the time constraints described below.

Limits on the number of attempts

Having passed the MCQ section, candidates must successfully complete the *whole* examination within 2 years from the date of their *first* attempt at the clinical section. Candidates may apply for an extension of this time limitation if there are valid extenuating circumstances (e.g. long-term illness, pregnancy, British Forces assignments).

The marking system

- A 1–5 marking scheme will be used for all sections:
  - — 5 = excellent pass
  - — 4 = good pass
  - — 3 = pass
  - — 2 = marginal fail
  - — 1 = fail
- The sections are independent of each other, although limited compensation may occur with each of the clinical and viva voce sections. Each section is thus given an equal weighting
- A 'pass' grade is needed for each MCQ paper
- In the clinical section, compensation between bays is possible. There are five examination bays and therefore five markings. The aggregate pass mark is 15. Examiners will discuss any candidate who is awarded a mark of 14 or who is awarded a mark of 1 in any section. A mark of 1 is only given under exceptional circumstances
- In the viva voce section compensation between vivas is possible. There are three vivas and therefore three markings. The aggregate pass mark is 9. Examiners will discuss any candidate who is awarded a mark of 8 or who is awarded a mark of 1 in any section. Again, a mark of 1 is only given under exceptional circumstances
- Examiners are in pairs for each section of the clinical and viva voce examination, which prevents any undue bias in marking.

Royal College of Surgeons of Edinburgh

The format for the AFRCS is almost identical to that for the MRCS awarded by the English College. It consists of:

The multiple-choice question papers
- MCQ 1: Principles of Surgery in General
- MCQ 2: Systematic Surgery.

Both MCQs may be taken at any time during the 2 years of basic surgical training and each paper will stand alone. There is no limit as to the number of times candidates may sit the papers. Both papers must be passed before a candidate may proceed to the final assessment.

The final assessment
This will consist of an oral and a clinical component and can be sat after a minimum of 20 months of basic surgical training.

- Orals (three in number)
  - critical care
  - principles of surgery including operative surgery and applied anatomy
  - clinical surgery and pathology based on the experience demonstrated in the candidate's log book
- Clinical
  - this covers the full range of specialties included in the syllabus
  - this lasts 40 minutes and during this time the candidate will see at least five clinical cases
  - this will be with two examiners
  - this examination will assess a candidate's ability to take an accurate history, elicit physical signs, produce a differential diagnosis and briefly discuss investigation and treatment.

Candidates *must* pass the final assessment within *2 years* of their first attempt at the oral examinations.

Royal College of Physicians and Surgeons of Glasgow

The examination again consists of two components:

The multiple-choice question papers
- These can be taken after a minimum of 9 months of basic surgical training
- There will be four 1-hour papers:
  - anatomy
  - physiology
  - pathology (including bacteriology)
  - clinical surgery
- All four papers will be held in one day

• Candidates must sit all the papers at the first sitting, but a pass in one or more of the papers may be carried forward to subsequent sittings of the MCQ papers until all four papers have been successfully passed.

The final assessment
This consists of an oral and a clinical section and trainees will not be eligible to sit these components of the examination until at least 18 months of Basic Surgical Training have been completed. There must be evidence of satisfactory clinical assessments and attendance at a Basic Surgical Skills course. The log book must be completed and verified by the candidate's surgical trainers.

The oral section
There will be two 30-minute orals in:

• Applied anatomy/operative surgery and principles and practice of surgery
• Applied physiology/bacteriology and critical care/surgical physiology.

The clinical section
• This will last 40 minutes and will consist of a 'ward round' situation in which the candidates will see a minimum of five patients of varying surgical specialties
• There will be two examiners
• This will assess the candidate's ability to elicit a concise history, demonstrate clinical findings and to appreciate the significance of clinical findings and appropriate management.

Candidates must achieve a minimum mark at the oral to proceed to the clinical. If this is 'marginal fail', the candidate will have to obtain additional marks in the clinical section to achieve a pass. Those candidates who fail to achieve an overall pass mark will be required to resit those sections of the examination that they have failed.

Royal College of Surgeons in Ireland

The examination consists of three parts:
• Multiple-choice questions
• Orals
• Clinical.

The multiple-choice questions

- There will be four 1-hour papers of 20 questions with five stems in each paper on the following subjects:
  — surgical anatomy
  — surgical physiology
  — applied pathology, microbiology and immunology
  — clinical surgery
- Each paper will have a total mark of 100, and to pass a candidate must attain an aggregate mark of 240.

The orals

- Only those who have passed the written paper are eligible to sit the oral examination
- The oral will consist of three 20-minute vivas on:
  — principles of operative surgery and surgical anatomy
  — critical care and surgical emergencies
  — principles of surgical management
- Each oral will be marked out of 100 and a candidate must achieve an aggregate mark of 180 to pass.

The clinical

- This will last for 1 hour and will be based on a minimum of five clinical cases
- Candidates will be required to take a history from one patient and to demonstrate the ability to elicit and interpret clinical signs
- There will be a variety of cases from differing surgical specialties.

Preparing for the examination

4

General comments

It is impossible to recommend a formal method of preparation for this examination that would suit all individuals. Furthermore, the emphasis today is far more on the entire educational package that a basic surgical trainee can participate in and experience, rather than the 'one-off' examination of yesteryear. Therefore, candidates for this examination should be better prepared than any of their predecessors in that they are now provided with a structured educational package, involving mandatory clinical training and the provision of a purpose-designed educational distance learning package in the form of the STEP course. However, there are certain practical ways in which a prospective candidate can improve his or her chances of success. This chapter could therefore be entitled: 'Surgical Common Sense — and How to Acquire It!'

1. A busy clinical surgical rotation in an environment where the senior staff are teaching-orientated is the best possible preparation for this examination. Most surgical rotations for BSTs should now provide such a facility.

2. Consistent, well-planned acquisition of surgical knowledge and expertise is far more profitable than a mad cram over the last few months. This is the advantage of a regular structured learning programme as provided by the STEP course and the staggered nature of the examination. It allows knowledge to be acquired in a stepwise manner and to be examined accordingly. It is therefore not necessarily best to take the two MCQ papers together, although individuals have the flexibility to proceed as suits them best. Furthermore, it is wise to start reading around the subjects and conditions as they present clinically on the wards right from the start of one's surgical career, as this broadens one's surgical horizons and gives a depth to surgical

understanding and experience. This is much better preparation than any amount of isolated sterile haphazard library work.

3. It is profitable to try to formulate a well-planned reading and revision programme that parallels the practical clinical experience being acquired during the various parts of a surgical rotation. For example, during the 6 months of orthopaedic surgery, acquire a practical textbook on the subject (see Appendix 3) and attempt to read a chapter a day. The daily clinical experience will then be supported by an ever-increasing depth of factual knowledge, while the planned reading programme will be enlivened by the recall of specific patients with the described clinical syndromes.

4. There will inevitably be gaps in clinical experience in that several major clinical specialties will not be covered within a limited 2-year programme. Courses like the STEP course seek to cover all aspects of the syllabus, and it is wise either to follow this or to be sure that the entire syllabus is covered in one's reading programme. Furthermore, it is invaluable to attend all teaching sessions provided by senior staff in the clinical subjects not covered in one's own rotation, as well as to take any opportunity that arises to examine patients in these other clinical specialties.

5. Ensure that your reading programme is varied and structured. There is nothing so boring, demoralizing and 'insomniac-curing' than to sit down with an enormous all-embracing surgical tome and attempt to read it from cover to cover in the final month before the clinical or viva voce examination. However, it is advisable to try to keep abreast of current surgical advances, and this is best achieved by 'dipping into' certain current journals. There is nothing that impresses an examiner more than a candidate who has actually read and understood relevant current articles. The following journals are worth looking at, not in depth, but for significant advances or valuable reviews:

- *British Journal of Surgery*
- *Annals of the Royal Colleges of Surgeons*
- *British Medical Journal* (especially leading articles and any surgical articles)
- *The Lancet* (leading articles)
- *Surgery* (especially designed review articles for teaching)
- *Hospital Doctor*
- *British Journal of Hospital Medicine* (review articles)
- Recently published texts on recent advances, etc.

6. Journal clubs and postgraduate meetings are of particular value and should be encouraged and used to keep abreast of current advances. Such meetings may initially tend to appear to be yet another rather boring meeting that an overworked BST has to attend. However, if they are well run, they can be a pleasant and modestly pain-free way of acquiring knowledge, as well as a useful forum in which the views of senior colleagues are aired and discussed. It is always valuable to take part or even just to listen to such discussion or debate, as the topics discussed can so often be asked during viva sessions.

7. Take every opportunity to practise presenting cases. This gives invaluable experience, not only in the examination of cases or looking up the relevant literature, but also in publicly marshalling your thought processes and speaking in public. It is much better to gain experience in being grilled over cases before a 'home crowd' rather than to wait until such 'grilling' is in earnest in front of a pair of examiners.

8. Take the opportunity wherever possible of taking part in formal teaching programmes such as the STEP course study days, or specifically designed courses. Any courses purposely meant for final revision before the clinical or viva examinations are extremely helpful, but are not meant for the first-time acquisition of knowledge. They are invaluable just prior to sitting the clinical part of the examination and aim to add polish to your examination technique and to tie up loose ends. Therefore, for maximum benefit only undertake them when sufficient clinical experience has been acquired, and this most probably means when both MCQ papers have been passed.

9. Seek to define any deficiencies in your knowledge. This can often be difficult, as few candidates have sufficient insight into their own inadequacies to define their own weak spots. Wise trainees will therefore seek the advice of their mentors or trainers to help them determine such deficiencies. It is pointless spending a great deal of time revising your strong points, although this is tempting, interesting and encouraging. Therefore, seek out any inadequacies and rectify them by a carefully planned revision and reading programme.

10. Do not take the examination too early. The colleges have indicated certain time restraints purposefully (see Ch. 3) and this is for the candidates' advantage as much as for any other reason. It is much better to take an examination when well prepared,

rather than to take it at the earliest feasible moment on the off chance that you might pass. This tactic seldom works and can be demoralizing. So prepare well, read widely, make the most of every clinical opportunity that presents itself, enrol on a formal BST training course such as the STEP course and follow College guidelines as to timing, and you will be as well prepared as any candidate can be.

The multiple-choice question papers

5

General comments

As outlined in Chapter 3, there are two multiple-choice question papers, each lasting 2 hours and based upon the modules of the syllabus as follows:

1. Core modules 1–5 (Principles of Surgery in General)
2. System modules A–E (Systematic Surgery).

These papers may be taken separately or at the same sitting; each paper will stand alone, and the candidate will be awarded either a 'pass' or 'fail' for each paper. Candidates may sit each of the MCQ papers as often as they wish. There is full reciprocity of recognition of a 'pass' in the MCQ section of the examination between all three UK surgical colleges and the Irish Surgical College. This chapter seeks to prepare the candidate for this part of the examination and give a little insight as to how these papers are prepared and what they seek to test in order for them to be answered most effectively.

Aims and content

The multiple-choice question papers seek to assess the candidate's knowledge in the following seven spheres:

- Factual knowledge
- Symptoms and signs
- Investigation with the correct sequencing
- Interpretation of results with emphasis on priorities
- Clinical management
- Prophylaxis and epidemiology
- Medicolegal issues.

Furthermore, it is proposed that the papers should contain not less than one third basic science-related questions to ensure that candidates have a grasp of such essential knowledge and are able to apply such knowledge. Questions will therefore test knowledge of basic science and clinical aspects, or a combination of both.

Attempts at question-spotting are futile, as an enormous bank of questions has been generated which is being continually added to. However, it is always wise to be aware of current issues and topical problems, as these inevitably tend to come to the front of the mind of a weary examiner attempting yet again to generate further questions for the bank.

MCQ papers are used to reliably and accurately test a candidate's depth of knowledge, and you will need to have detailed knowledge in order to pass. As this is the most structured part of the examination, it aims to test knowledge of a precise nature, both as to subject-matter and as to finer detail.

Format of the MCQ papers

Each college publishes details as to the format of its MCQ paper. For the Royal College of Surgeons of England each paper is subdivided into two sections:

- Multiple true-false questions
- Extended matching questions.

The college sends candidates advice sheets in advance to allow familiarity with the style of questions before the actual examination. Take time to familiarize yourself with these two forms of question. Examples of each form are given below.

Multiple true-false questions

This is the simplest form of multiple-choice question, in which a stem provides a focus for a group of about three to seven statements that are either 'true' or 'false'. The stem is usually brief, announcing the subject-matter which may be a disease, an organ or a condition. The group of true-false items tend to have a coherence rather than be a disparate group of unrelated topics.

Every attempt is made in formulating the questions to avoid any ambiguity or lack of clarity. Vague terms are avoided and, in order to prevent any controversy as to the precise intended meaning of any particular term, a glossary of terminology is provided with each paper (see Appendix 2). Furthermore, accepted abbreviations are also printed with the paper (see Appendix 1).

It is important to note that *all* or *none* of the options may be true, or any number in between.

It is vital not just to mark those which are true, but also to mark the paper with those that are false.

Examples of multiple true-false questions

Core module questions

1. The right adrenal gland:
    - x A   is separated from the liver by the hepatorenal recess
    - x B   has venous drainage to the right renal vein
    - x C   lies in front of the inferior vena cava
    - x D   is usually exposed during right nephrectomy for non-malignant causes
    - ✓ E   has the diaphragm as a posterior relation

2. Local anaesthetics:
    - x A   act better on large nerve fibres than small
    - ✓ B   work by blocking the Na channels
    - x C   are all vasoconstrictors
    - x D   are ineffective topically
    - x E   stimulate the generation of action potentials

System module questions

1. The following conditions can cause Raynaud's phenomenon:
    - ✓ A   frost bite
    - ✓ B   scleroderma
    - ✓ C   vibrating tools
    - ✓ D   polycythaemia
    - x E   leukaemia
    - x F   hyperthyroidism

2. Thyroid cancer is:
    - x A   more common in males than females
    - ✓ B   a complication of irradiation therapy after a latent period of 15 years
    - x C   the commonest cause of SVC obstruction
    - x D   particularly aggressive in young patients
    - ✓ E   accountable for 10–30% of clinically solitary nodules that are resected

The answer sheet for the above two system modules multiple true-false questions is shown in Figure 5.1.

A	B	C	D	E	F	G	H
1 [T] [F]	[T] [F]	[T] [F]	[T] [F]	[T] [F]	[T] [F]	[T] [F]	[T] [F]
2 [T] [F]	[T] [F]	[T] [F]	[T] [F]	[T] [F]	[T] [F]	[T] [F]	[T] [F]

Example of answers correctly coded on exam sheet

Fig. 5.1 Answer sheet for example of system modules multiple true-false questions.

Extended matching questions

These questions are designed to test more than simple factual knowledge, and seek to assess the application of knowledge, priorities and good practice.

Each question will be headed by a theme, or short title, designed to focus attention on the subject-matter. This will then be followed by a list of up to 10 options which will be the possible answers to the questions or clinical vignettes that appear subsequently. After the option list there is a sentence asking the candidate to pick the most likely option from the list to fit the descriptions given, stressing that each option may be used *once, more than once* or *not at all* for the whole question. However, each description will only have one correct answer or option that applies to it. Each description listed may describe a clinical situation, an investigation or some other scenario for which one of the options given will be the most appropriate response.

It is clearly stated in the English College paper that marks will not be deducted for a wrong answer, but equally you will not gain a mark if you mark more than one option.

Examples of extended matching questions

Core modules
Theme: Nipple discharge

Options:
A Cyclical discharge
B Breast abscess
C Sclerosing adenosis
D Duct ectasia   (1)
E Galactorrhoea
F Duct papilloma   (2)

For each of the patients described below, select the *single* most likely diagnosis from the list of options above. Each option may be used once, more than once or not at all.

1. A 45-year-old woman complains of a discharge from her right nipple. On examination she is found to have a creamy discharge from multiple duct orifices on the right nipple, which is retracted, and a firm, subareolar mass is palpated on that side. The nipple discharge is positive on testing for blood.

2. A 40-year-old woman presents with a frankly blood-stained discharge from her left nipple. The discharge is seen to emerge from a single duct orifice. Bilateral breast and axillary examination is otherwise normal.

System modules
Theme: Adrenal lesions

Options:

A Adrenal cortical hyperplasia	(65)
B Phaeochromocytoma	
C Adrenogenital syndrome	
D Conn's syndrome	
E Addison's disease	
F Neuroblastoma	(66)

For each of the patients described below select the *single* most likely diagnosis from the list of options above. Each option may be used once, more than once, or not at all.

65. A 46-year-old woman who has smoked 15 cigarettes a day for several years presents with a productive cough, headache, amenorrhoea, weakness and lethargy. She has a round, plethoric face with acne and facial hair. She has striae on her protruberant abdominal wall and her BP is 190/110 mmHg.

66. An 8-month-old male infant presenting with proptosis of the right eye, abdominal distension and failure to thrive is found to have a balotable left-sided abdominal mass.

The answer sheet for the above system module extended matching questions (65 & 66) is shown in Figure 5.2.

	A	**B**	**C**	**D**	**E**	**F**	**G**	**H**	**I**	**J**
65	[A]	[B]	[C]	[D]	[E]	[F]	[G]	[H]	[I]	[J]
66	[A]	[B]	[C]	[D]	[E]	[F]	[G]	[H]	[I]	[J]

Example of answers correctly coded on exam sheet

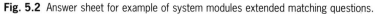

Fig. 5.2 Answer sheet for example of system modules extended matching questions.

Note: For each of the above questions, no option was used twice, but this is not to be taken for granted, and there may be questions when one particular option is correct for more than one clinical vignette. However, each vignette has only one correct answer from the list of options.

Preparing for the MCQ papers

1. Practise answering multiple-choice questions. There is a large variety of MCQ books on the market and several are already published that are geared towards this examination.
2. MCQ practice will also increase your basic knowledge and most such books now explain the answers given. This method also makes for far more interesting revision. It is particularly productive to practise MCQs relating to the subject that is the current topic of your revision programme, as this serves to further reinforce your knowledge.
3. Do not try to 'question spot' or to attempt to remember hundreds of isolated or dislocated facts. It is far more profitable to seek to understand your subject and thus be able to apply good surgical principles to the problems presented.
4. Find out what marking scheme is being used for whichever examination is being sat — e.g. the Royal College of Surgeons of England does not use negative marking, following the example of the Royal College of General Practitioners. This means that a neutral marking system is employed in which no marks are subtracted for incorrect responses. In this form of marking there is no disadvantage to guessing, and it is to your advantage not to leave any questions unanswered as you will lose marks. Even with complete guessing, it is likely that by random chance alone you will gain 50%, but this assumes that there are an equal number of 'true' and 'false' answers, and this is by no means to be taken for granted. However, if you have a good understanding of the subject, it means that it is well worth while following your 'inclination' when undertaking an examination using neutral marking. If negative marking is being used, this means that a mark is deducted for every wrong answer given. Therefore, in this form of examination a blind guess is not necessarily the best practice. It may be wise in this context to practise several MCQ papers to try and assess whether your 'inclination' answers actually provide you with a good score or an inferior score. If too many answers rely upon your 'inclination' or too many are wrong, then this suggests that you are not ready to

sit this part of the examination. It may appear that neutral marking is a softer option than negative marking, but this is not necessarily true. Indeed, the marking method is taken into account in setting pass marks, and some studies have shown neutral marking to be a better discriminator.

5. Do ensure that you fully understand the instructions issued by the respective Royal Colleges regarding this part of the examination. Full details and sheets entitled 'Advice to Candidates on the Multiple Choice Question Papers' are available from the Examinations Department. This provides clear details as to the nature of the paper, sample questions, as listed above, a glossary of terms and abbreviations and examples of the instruction sheets that will be issued to the candidate along with the actual paper on examination day.

Sitting the MCQ papers

1. As with every examination paper, *read the instructions carefully*. All too many candidates have failed examinations in the past because they have failed to follow this simple advice and have either answered the wrong question, presented it incorrectly, not taken account of the time allowed or not presented their answer in an appropriate manner. Do not fall into this trap, but read the paper instructions carefully and twice, and then follow them religiously.

2. Be sure to enter your candidate number in the prescribed way (see Fig. 5.3). You may have performed outstandingly, but if nobody can identify you, you will receive no credit for your labours.

3. Do be sure to apportion your time correctly. In the English College paper it is recommended that you spend $1^1/_4$ hours on section 1, which includes the multiple true-false questions, and $^3/_4$ hour on section 2, which includes the extended matching questions. Do ensure that you do not run out of time.

4. Look carefully at the answer sheet provided. Remember it will be marked optically, so do not put any mark on the paper other than those specifically related to your intended answers. In this respect you will most probably be given a special pencil with which to mark your paper; if so, *use it*, and do *not* use any other pen, ballpoint or ordinary pencil.

5. Do not fold or crease your answer sheet or in any way deface it, as this may make it impossible to be marked optically. Any sheet that is marked in any way other than that prescribed may well be rejected by the computer.

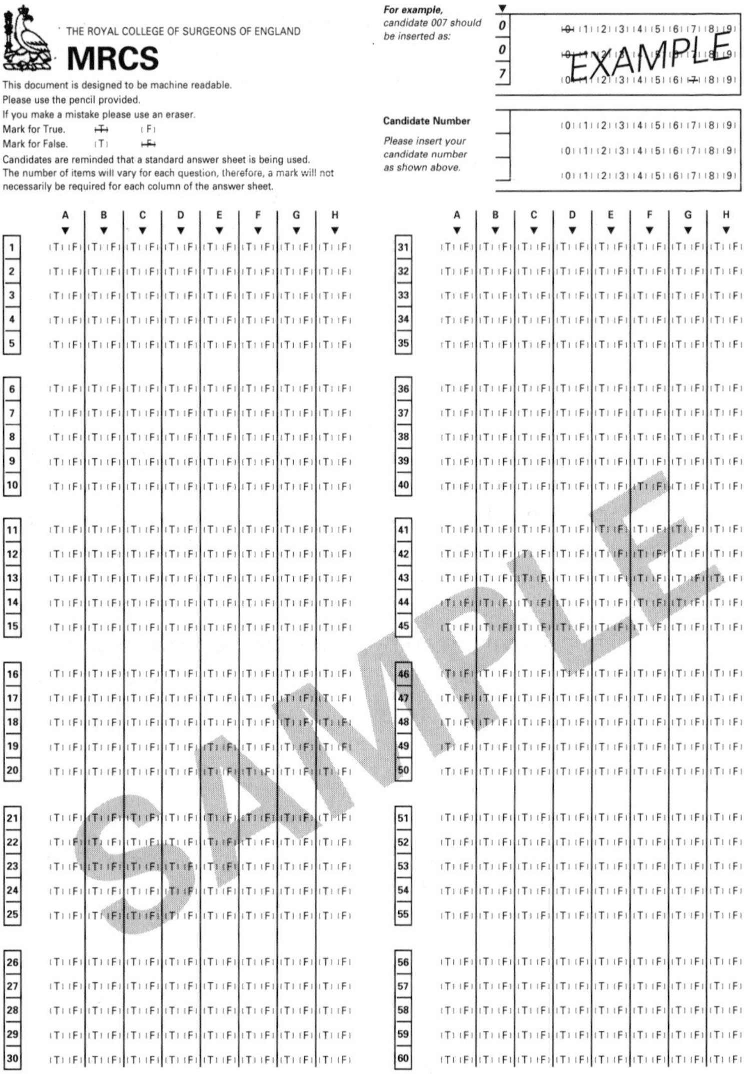

THE ROYAL COLLEGE OF SURGEONS OF ENGLAND

MRCS

This document is designed to be machine readable.
Please use the pencil provided.
If you make a mistake please use an eraser.
Mark for True. (T) (F)
Mark for False. (T) (F)
Candidates are reminded that a standard answer sheet is being used.
The number of items will vary for each question, therefore, a mark will not necessarily be required for each column of the answer sheet.

For example, candidate 007 should be inserted as:

0	(0) (1) (2) (3) (4) (5) (6) (7) (8) (9)
0	(0) (1) (2) (3) (4) (5) (6) (7) (8) (9)
7	(0) (1) (2) (3) (4) (5) (6) (7) (8) (9)

EXAMPLE

Candidate Number

Please insert your candidate number as shown above.

	(0) (1) (2) (3) (4) (5) (6) (7) (8) (9)
	(0) (1) (2) (3) (4) (5) (6) (7) (8) (9)
	(0) (1) (2) (3) (4) (5) (6) (7) (8) (9)

	A	B	C	D	E	F	G	H
1	(T) (F)	(T) (F)	(T) (F)	(T) (F)	(T) (F)	(T) (F)	(T) (F)	(T) (F)
2	(T) (F)	(T) (F)	(T) (F)	(T) (F)	(T) (F)	(T) (F)	(T) (F)	(T) (F)
3	(T) (F)	(T) (F)	(T) (F)	(T) (F)	(T) (F)	(T) (F)	(T) (F)	(T) (F)
4	(T) (F)	(T) (F)	(T) (F)	(T) (F)	(T) (F)	(T) (F)	(T) (F)	(T) (F)
5	(T) (F)	(T) (F)	(T) (F)	(T) (F)	(T) (F)	(T) (F)	(T) (F)	(T) (F)
6	(T) (F)	(T) (F)	(T) (F)	(T) (F)	(T) (F)	(T) (F)	(T) (F)	(T) (F)
7	(T) (F)	(T) (F)	(T) (F)	(T) (F)	(T) (F)	(T) (F)	(T) (F)	(T) (F)
8	(T) (F)	(T) (F)	(T) (F)	(T) (F)	(T) (F)	(T) (F)	(T) (F)	(T) (F)
9	(T) (F)	(T) (F)	(T) (F)	(T) (F)	(T) (F)	(T) (F)	(T) (F)	(T) (F)
10	(T) (F)	(T) (F)	(T) (F)	(T) (F)	(T) (F)	(T) (F)	(T) (F)	(T) (F)
11	(T) (F)	(T) (F)	(T) (F)	(T) (F)	(T) (F)	(T) (F)	(T) (F)	(T) (F)
12	(T) (F)	(T) (F)	(T) (F)	(T) (F)	(T) (F)	(T) (F)	(T) (F)	(T) (F)
13	(T) (F)	(T) (F)	(T) (F)	(T) (F)	(T) (F)	(T) (F)	(T) (F)	(T) (F)
14	(T) (F)	(T) (F)	(T) (F)	(T) (F)	(T) (F)	(T) (F)	(T) (F)	(T) (F)
15	(T) (F)	(T) (F)	(T) (F)	(T) (F)	(T) (F)	(T) (F)	(T) (F)	(T) (F)
16	(T) (F)	(T) (F)	(T) (F)	(T) (F)	(T) (F)	(T) (F)	(T) (F)	(T) (F)
17	(T) (F)	(T) (F)	(T) (F)	(T) (F)	(T) (F)	(T) (F)	(T) (F)	(T) (F)
18	(T) (F)	(T) (F)	(T) (F)	(T) (F)	(T) (F)	(T) (F)	(T) (F)	(T) (F)
19	(T) (F)	(T) (F)	(T) (F)	(T) (F)	(T) (F)	(T) (F)	(T) (F)	(T) (F)
20	(T) (F)	(T) (F)	(T) (F)	(T) (F)	(T) (F)	(T) (F)	(T) (F)	(T) (F)
21	(T) (F)	(T) (F)	(T) (F)	(T) (F)	(T) (F)	(T) (F)	(T) (F)	(T) (F)
22	(T) (F)	(T) (F)	(T) (F)	(T) (F)	(T) (F)	(T) (F)	(T) (F)	(T) (F)
23	(T) (F)	(T) (F)	(T) (F)	(T) (F)	(T) (F)	(T) (F)	(T) (F)	(T) (F)
24	(T) (F)	(T) (F)	(T) (F)	(T) (F)	(T) (F)	(T) (F)	(T) (F)	(T) (F)
25	(T) (F)	(T) (F)	(T) (F)	(T) (F)	(T) (F)	(T) (F)	(T) (F)	(T) (F)
26	(T) (F)	(T) (F)	(T) (F)	(T) (F)	(T) (F)	(T) (F)	(T) (F)	(T) (F)
27	(T) (F)	(T) (F)	(T) (F)	(T) (F)	(T) (F)	(T) (F)	(T) (F)	(T) (F)
28	(T) (F)	(T) (F)	(T) (F)	(T) (F)	(T) (F)	(T) (F)	(T) (F)	(T) (F)
29	(T) (F)	(T) (F)	(T) (F)	(T) (F)	(T) (F)	(T) (F)	(T) (F)	(T) (F)
30	(T) (F)	(T) (F)	(T) (F)	(T) (F)	(T) (F)	(T) (F)	(T) (F)	(T) (F)

	A	B	C	D	E	F	G	H
31	(T) (F)	(T) (F)	(T) (F)	(T) (F)	(T) (F)	(T) (F)	(T) (F)	(T) (F)
32	(T) (F)	(T) (F)	(T) (F)	(T) (F)	(T) (F)	(T) (F)	(T) (F)	(T) (F)
33	(T) (F)	(T) (F)	(T) (F)	(T) (F)	(T) (F)	(T) (F)	(T) (F)	(T) (F)
34	(T) (F)	(T) (F)	(T) (F)	(T) (F)	(T) (F)	(T) (F)	(T) (F)	(T) (F)
35	(T) (F)	(T) (F)	(T) (F)	(T) (F)	(T) (F)	(T) (F)	(T) (F)	(T) (F)
36	(T) (F)	(T) (F)	(T) (F)	(T) (F)	(T) (F)	(T) (F)	(T) (F)	(T) (F)
37	(T) (F)	(T) (F)	(T) (F)	(T) (F)	(T) (F)	(T) (F)	(T) (F)	(T) (F)
38	(T) (F)	(T) (F)	(T) (F)	(T) (F)	(T) (F)	(T) (F)	(T) (F)	(T) (F)
39	(T) (F)	(T) (F)	(T) (F)	(T) (F)	(T) (F)	(T) (F)	(T) (F)	(T) (F)
40	(T) (F)	(T) (F)	(T) (F)	(T) (F)	(T) (F)	(T) (F)	(T) (F)	(T) (F)
41	(T) (F)	(T) (F)	(T) (F)	(T) (F)	(T) (F)	(T) (F)	(T) (F)	(T) (F)
42	(T) (F)	(T) (F)	(T) (F)	(T) (F)	(T) (F)	(T) (F)	(T) (F)	(T) (F)
43	(T) (F)	(T) (F)	(T) (F)	(T) (F)	(T) (F)	(T) (F)	(T) (F)	(T) (F)
44	(T) (F)	(T) (F)	(T) (F)	(T) (F)	(T) (F)	(T) (F)	(T) (F)	(T) (F)
45	(T) (F)	(T) (F)	(T) (F)	(T) (F)	(T) (F)	(T) (F)	(T) (F)	(T) (F)
46	(T) (F)	(T) (F)	(T) (F)	(T) (F)	(T) (F)	(T) (F)	(T) (F)	(T) (F)
47	(T) (F)	(T) (F)	(T) (F)	(T) (F)	(T) (F)	(T) (F)	(T) (F)	(T) (F)
48	(T) (F)	(T) (F)	(T) (F)	(T) (F)	(T) (F)	(T) (F)	(T) (F)	(T) (F)
49	(T) (F)	(T) (F)	(T) (F)	(T) (F)	(T) (F)	(T) (F)	(T) (F)	(T) (F)
50	(T) (F)	(T) (F)	(T) (F)	(T) (F)	(T) (F)	(T) (F)	(T) (F)	(T) (F)
51	(T) (F)	(T) (F)	(T) (F)	(T) (F)	(T) (F)	(T) (F)	(T) (F)	(T) (F)
52	(T) (F)	(T) (F)	(T) (F)	(T) (F)	(T) (F)	(T) (F)	(T) (F)	(T) (F)
53	(T) (F)	(T) (F)	(T) (F)	(T) (F)	(T) (F)	(T) (F)	(T) (F)	(T) (F)
54	(T) (F)	(T) (F)	(T) (F)	(T) (F)	(T) (F)	(T) (F)	(T) (F)	(T) (F)
55	(T) (F)	(T) (F)	(T) (F)	(T) (F)	(T) (F)	(T) (F)	(T) (F)	(T) (F)
56	(T) (F)	(T) (F)	(T) (F)	(T) (F)	(T) (F)	(T) (F)	(T) (F)	(T) (F)
57	(T) (F)	(T) (F)	(T) (F)	(T) (F)	(T) (F)	(T) (F)	(T) (F)	(T) (F)
58	(T) (F)	(T) (F)	(T) (F)	(T) (F)	(T) (F)	(T) (F)	(T) (F)	(T) (F)
59	(T) (F)	(T) (F)	(T) (F)	(T) (F)	(T) (F)	(T) (F)	(T) (F)	(T) (F)
60	(T) (F)	(T) (F)	(T) (F)	(T) (F)	(T) (F)	(T) (F)	(T) (F)	(T) (F)

Fig. 5.3 Facsimile of MCQ answer sheet.

6. Marks will only be awarded for answers clearly entered on the provided answer sheet. No other method of scoring is allowed.
7. Do not attempt to try and calculate how many answers you will need to provide. The number of questions that the candidate is expected to answer will vary from paper to paper, as will the proportion of 'true' to 'false' answers.

8. You may find it safer to go through the paper answering the questions in your question booklet and subsequently transferring your marks to the computer-marked answer sheet. Indeed, it is recommended that you:

- Transfer marks after completion of each section separately
  This will prove less confusing. Therefore complete the multiple true-false section first, noting that you will have approximately $1^1/_4$ hours in which to complete it.
- Consider each question and mark your answer book with a 'tick' or 'cross' depending on whether you consider an answer 'true' or 'false' for the multiple true-false questions. Then transfer your answers to the answer sheet using the technique advised.
- Ensure that you allow time to transfer your marks across to the computer-marked answer sheet. Your marked question book will *not* be acceptable.
- Now complete the extended matching question section, marking your question booklet with your preferred option for each question. Then transfer your answers to the answer sheet.
- It must be stressed once more that sufficient time must be allowed to transfer your marks onto the official answer sheet. No additional time will be allowed at the end of the examination to transfer the marks.

Finally...

Multiple-choice question papers can be fun as long as you obey the rules. Therefore, the golden rules of MCQ papers are:

- Read the instructions
- Follow the instructions
- Insert your number
- Watch the time
- Fill in the answer sheet accurately.

The clinical examination

6

The format of the clinical examination

The format of the clinical examination for each of the differing surgical colleges varies slightly as laid out in Chapter 3. In order to provide a flavour of this part of the examination, the format of the examination as conducted by the English College will be described in detail, but the principles applied will be identical for all the colleges. All will consist of short cases covering a variety of surgical specialities. In the English College each candidate will visit five bays in which the following cases are likely to be seen:

- Bay 1: Superficial lesions
- Bay 2: Musculoskeletal and neurological cases
- Bay 3: Circulatory and lymphatic cases
- Bay 4: The abdomen and trunk
- Bay 5: Communication skills.

For further details of the types of cases in each bay and how they should be approached see Chapters 7–11.

General hints for the clinical examination

1. Never fabricate or exaggerate any clinical symptoms or signs as the examiner will immediately label you as an unreliable witness and poor clinician.
2. In order to prepare for this aspect of the examination, take every opportunity at your own hospital to present cases in public. Initially it can be a traumatic experience, but it is far better to practise your technique of presentation in front of a supportive home audience, rather than for the first time in the more critical situation across the green baize table. Therefore, practise presenting cases clearly and concisely, choosing the important features that need to be emphasized.

3. Always use surgical terminology to describe your findings and be as precise as possible.
4. Accurately locate symptoms or signs. For example:
   - For the abdomen:
     — epigastrium
     — hypochondrium
     — periumbilical
     — loins
     — flank
     — iliac fossae
     — hypogastrium or suprapubic
   - For the chest:
     — upper, mid or lower zone
     — mid-clavicular, anterior and posterior axillary lines
   - Planes:
     — coronal
     — sagittal
   - Paired terminology:
     — supine or prone
     — supination or pronation
     — dorsal or ventral
     — valgus or varus
     — medial or lateral (median)
     — proximal or distal
     — cephalic or caudal
     — afferent or efferent
5. Take your own stethoscope to the clinical part of the examination, but all other essential equipment will be provided for you. However, to save time, it is wise to also take a tape measure, pocket torch, tongue spatula, and possibly a disposable glove for examination of the mouth (rectal and vaginal examinations are not permitted). These articles will help prevent a queue at the equipment table.
6. Much of the content of the next five chapters may be found in greater depth in many standard textbooks (Appendix 3), but it is included for completeness and to assist the candidate in his or her preparation and presentation.

The examination

The purpose of this part of the examination is to assess the clinical examination technique of the candidate, as well as his or her ability to interpret clinical findings.

It is important to realize that this session is not a race against time, and marks will usually be awarded for quality and not simply quantity. Remember that the examiner will be concentrating on the candidate's ability to elicit clinical signs, interpret them and come to a reasoned plan of management.

Always treat your patient as an individual, and not simply as another case. Be careful *never* to hurt the patient — you are seeking to convince the examiner that you are a kind, compassionate and discerning clinician and hurting the patient will not further this cause. Therefore always be gentle. It often pays to ask the patient whether the lesion, etc., is tender prior to examining it.

Present your findings clearly and simply, and do not include irrelevancies. You do not want to waste time discussing what a lesion is not, but try and concentrate on the positive features.

Do *not* cut corners. Always examine the patient properly and do not skimp on your technique because you are in an examination. Many candidates fail by jumping to illogical conclusions, or by forsaking first principles when it comes to examining common lesions such as herniae. Make sure all your patients are examined thoroughly and efficiently.

Describe what you see and feel. You may not always be able to reach a definite diagnosis, but by accurately describing the physical signs, you should be able to formulate a plan for investigation or treatment.

Do not panic if you do not know what a lesion is (Fig. 6.1). It is possible that the examiner may not know what it is either. Such cases are often included as they make good discussion points.

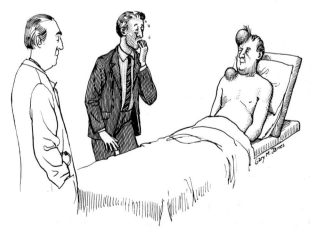

Fig. 6.1 'Do *not* panic.'

If your physical signs are wrong, and the examiner points this out, try and accept the situation with cheerful humility. You should aim to give the impression of being suitably fascinated by this interesting physical sign.

Some golden rules for short cases

The types of cases will be so varied that it is difficult to give specific hints. However, the following factors apply to whatever major system is affected.

1. Do not forget to observe the patient's general facies, demeanour and nutritional state. The best time to assess these is when you first meet him or her. The moment you are introduced to the patient, consider whether there are any abnormalities in the facies or general appearance.
   - Is the patient jaundiced, anaemic, cyanosed?
   - Is the patient dehydrated, cachectic, obese?
   - What about the facial expression?
   - Is the patient in pain?
   - Is there a facial palsy?
   - Are there any features of classical syndromes? For example,
     — myxoedema
     — thyrotoxicosis
     — acromegaly (Fig. 6.2)
     — Cushing's syndrome
     — Addison's disease
     — myasthenia gravis
     — polycythaemia
     — neurofibromatosis
     — carcinoid syndrome (flushing)
   - Are there any drips, tubes, drains, etc., which might provide valuable clues?
2. Opportunity usually arises to ask the patient a few specific questions while you are carrying out your examination. However, make sure that the questions are relevant to the lesion being examined, and that they do not detract from your examination technique.
3. The patient's eyes, hands, tongue and pulse can often give valuable clues as to their general health. Do not forget to look for:
   - Eyes: exophthalmos (Fig. 6.3), pupil size (e.g. Horner's syndrome, Fig. 6.4), ptosis, arcus senilis, jaundiced sclera
   - Hands: clubbing (Fig. 6.5), koilonychia, leuconychia, liver palms, Heberden's nodes, muscle wasting, Dupuytren's contracture (Fig. 6.6), deformities, arachnodactyl (Fig. 6.7)

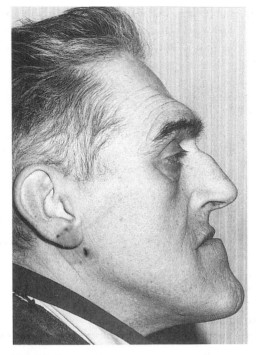

Fig. 6.2 Acromegaly.

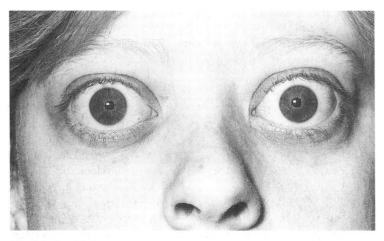

Fig. 6.3 Exophthalmos.

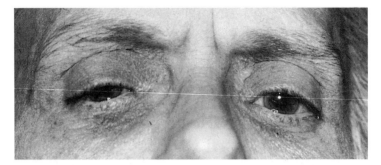

Fig. 6.4 Horner's syndrome.

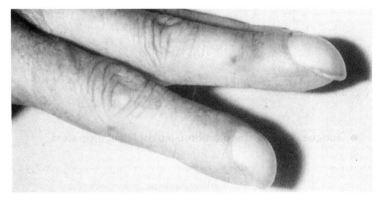

Fig. 6.5 Clubbing.

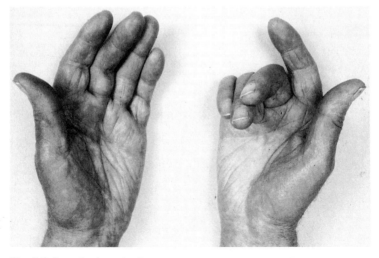

Fig. 6.6 Dupuytren's contracture.

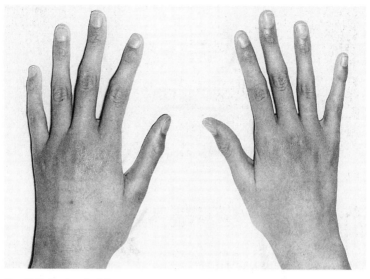

Fig. 6.7 Arachnodactyl.

- Tongue: furring, discoloration, leukoplakia, ulceration
- Pulse: rate, rhythm, character.
4. Always compare the diseased or injured side, limb, member or organ with its opposite healthy number. For example:
   - The breast
     — its shape
     — its size
     — its nipple
     — its skin dimpling
   - The pupil
     — its size
     — its reaction
   - The groin
     — any swellings
     — any cough impulse
     — any further herniae
   - The limbs. Assess for any difference in:
     — oedema
     — temperature
     — colour
     — wasting
     — localized swelling
     — deformity.

Clinical bay 1: Superficial lesions

7

In this bay you may expect to be shown lesions such as:

- Lipomata (Fig. 7.1)
- Sebaceous/epidermoid cysts (Fig. 7.2)
- Lymph nodes
- Benign and malignant skin lesions (Fig. 7.3)
- Other connective tissue lesions such as neurofibromata
- Salivary gland swellings (Fig. 7.4)
- Branchial cysts and sinuses (Fig. 7.5)
- Cervical ribs
- Thyroid swellings (Fig. 7.6)
- Breast lesions
- Ganglia
- Ingrowing toenails
- Onychogryphosis (Fig. 7.7).

You may be asked to comment on relevant scans, X-rays or pathology reports. Approach each case as you would in outpatients

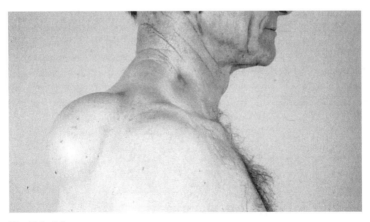

Fig. 7.1 A lipoma.

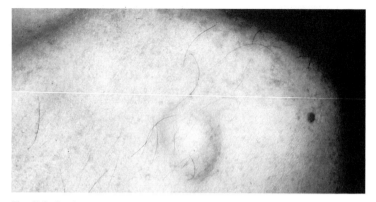

Fig. 7.2 A sebaceous cyst.

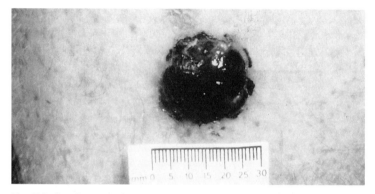

Fig. 7.3 A malignant melanoma.

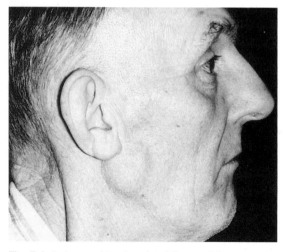

Fig. 7.4 A pleomorphic adenoma of the parotid.

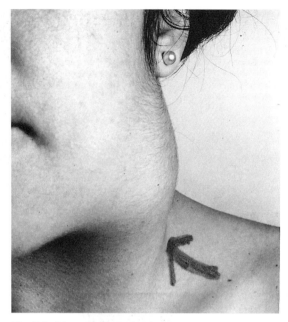

Fig. 7.5 A branchial cyst.

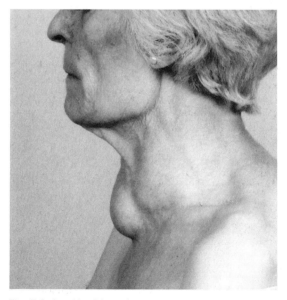

Fig. 7.6 A multinodular goitre.

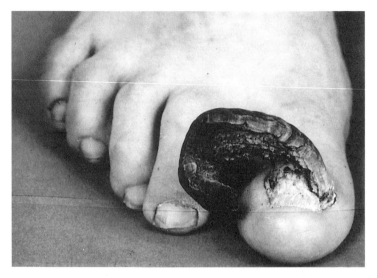

Fig. 7.7 Onychogryphosis.

Lumps

Always describe lumps in the following manner:

1. Site
   - The anatomical position including the side
   - The anatomical plane, e.g. is it in the:
     — skin
     — subcutaneous tissue
     — muscle
     — tendon
     — nerve
     — bone?
2. Size: measure it in cm.
3. Shape: is it:
   - round
   - flat
   - irregular
   - bosselated?
4. Skin: is the skin over it:
   - normal
   - thinned

- ulcerated
- fixed
- containing dilated veins?
5. Edge: is it:
   - distinct
   - indistinct
   - irregular?
6. Consistency: is it:
   - soft
   - firm
   - hard
   - bone hard
   - fluctuant
   - pulsatile?
7. Fixity: is it fixed to:
   - skin
   - muscle
   - bone
   - some deeper organ?
8. Other factors
   - Is it:
     — discoloured
     — tender
     — warm
     — reducible
     — indentable (e.g. faeces and some large dermoid cysts)?
   - Does it:
     — empty (e.g. cavernous haemangioma)
     — have a bruit
     — transilluminate?
   - State of:
     — adjacent tissues
     — regional lymph nodes
     — local circulation
     — local innervation
     — bones and joints?

Testing for fluctuation

Test by applying intermittent pressure with the index finger of one hand, between two fingers of the other hand (Fig. 7.8). This should be done in two planes at right angles to each other.

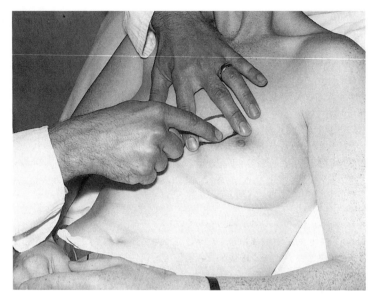

Fig. 7.8 Testing for fluctuation.

Testing for pulsation

Test by applying your fingers to either side of the lesion. A pulsatile lesion will expand in two dimensions, while a mass that is simply transmitting pulsation will not.

Ulcers

Always describe ulcers in the following manner:

1. Site: the anatomical position and side, for example:
   - rodent ulcers on the upper part of the face
   - carcinoma on the lower lip
   - primary chancre on the upper lip.
2. Number: single or multiple.
3. Size: measure it in cm.
4. Shape: is it:
   - circular
   - oval
   - irregular
   - serpiginous (healing in one place while extending in another — likened to a creeping serpent)?

5. Edge: is it:
   - shelved (e.g. varicose ulcer)
   - everted (e.g. carcinoma)
   - rolled or raised (e.g. rodent ulcer)
   - undermined (e.g. tuberculous ulcer)
   - punched-out (e.g. syphilitic ulcer)?
6. Floor: is it:
   - slough
   - watery
   - healthy granulation tissue
   - irregular tumour?
7. Base: is it:
   - indurated
   - attached to deeper structures
   - associated with an underlying mass?
8. Surrounding skin: is it:
   - inflamed
   - pigmented
   - telangiectatic
   - ischaemic
   - associated with varicosities?
9. Discharge: is it:
   - pus
   - bloodstained
   - watery
   - coloured (blue-green with *Pseudomonas*)?
10. Pain: is it:
    - tender
    - non-tender (e.g. primary chancre)?
11. Lymphatic drainage: is there any evidence of:
    - lymphadenopathy
    - lymphangitis?
12. Adjacent tissues
    - local circulation
    - local innervation
    - bones and joints.

Lymph nodes

Causes of enlargement:

- Infective
  - non-specific

— glandular fever
— tuberculosis
— toxoplasmosis
— syphilis
— cat scratch fever
— lymphogranuloma
— filariasis
- Metastatic tumour
- Reticulosis
  — non-Hodgkin's lymphoma
  — Hodgkin's disease
- Sarcoidosis.

Neck swellings

1. Number: single or multiple.
2. Site: anterior or posterior triangle.
3. Consistency: solid or cystic.
4. Movement:
   - with swallowing
   - with protrusion of tongue
   - no movement with either.
5. Classification
   - Multiple lumps: lymph nodes
   - Single lumps in the posterior triangle
     — not moving
       — solid: lymph node
       — cystic
         — cystic hygroma
         — pharyngeal pouch
       — pulsatile: aneurysm
   - Single lumps in the anterior triangle
     — not moving
       — solid
         — lymph node
         — carotid body tumour (transmits pulsation)
       — cystic
         — branchial cyst
         — cold abscess
     — moving with swallowing
       — solid: thyroid nodule
       — cystic: thyroid cyst

— moving with tongue protrusion
  — solid: thyroglossal ectopic thyroid tissue
  — cystic: thryoglossal cyst.

The thyroid

Inspection

- Sit opposite the patient in a good light.
- Don't forget to carefully assess the patient's general demeanour, face and eyes.
  For example, is there any sign of:
  — myxoedema
    — mental slowness
    — poorly marked outer eyebrows
    — dry, scanty and coarse hair
    — puffiness of the eyelids
    — a burgundy malar flush
    — a slow 'worn-out' voice?
  — thyrotoxicosis
    — nervous tension
    — fine tremor
    — exophthalmos (see below)
    — lid lag
    — signs of weight loss?
  — A retrosternal thyroid causing thoracic inlet obstruction
    — respiratory stridor
    — dilated veins?
- Look for specific features of an enlarged thyroid gland
  — Is there an obvious goitre? (Fig. 7.6) Is it bilateral or unilateral?
  — Give the patient a glass of water and ask them to swallow
  — Thyroid swellings (because of the attachment of the thyroid gland to the larynx/trachea by the ligament of Berry and because of its inclusion within the pretrachial fascia) will move upwards on swallowing, unless fixed by malignant infiltration or active inflammation
  — A thyroglossal cyst will move on protruding the tongue
  — Look for any pattern of enlargement. Is it:
    — regular
    — irregular
    — bosselated?

Palpation

- Do this from behind (Fig. 7.9)
- Relax the strap muscles by getting the patient to slightly lower their chin
- Palpate both lobes of the gland and the isthmus with the fingers of both hands, while the thumbs rest on the nape of the neck
- Define the extents of the gland, requesting the patient to swallow again
- Is the gland uniformly enlarged? If so, is it:
  — smooth
  — multinodular
  — hard
  — firm?
- Does the gland contain any discrete swellings or solitary nodules? If so, is it:
  — cystic
  — solid
  — a dominant nodule in a multinodular goitre?

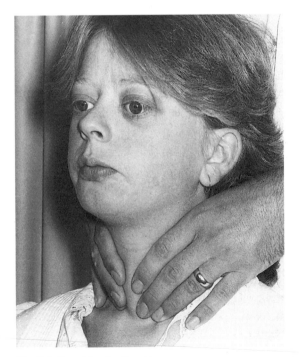

Fig. 7.9 Examining the thyroid.

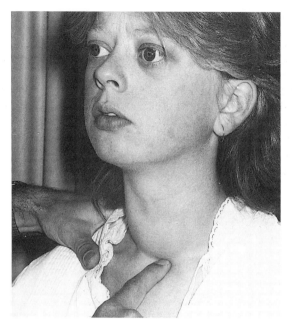

Fig. 7.10 Assessing for tracheal deviation.

- Does the swelling extend retrosternally?
- Is the trachea deviated (Fig. 7.10)? (This is usually better assessed from in front by placing your finger in the suprasternal notch.)
- Is the gland fixed, suggesting malignancy, and are there any lymph nodes palpable?
- Is there a thyroid thrill? (Only present in very advanced cases of thyrotoxicosis.)

Percussion

Some surgeons find it helpful to percuss for any retrosternal extension (not a very sensitive physical sign).

Auscultation

Toxic thyroids often exhibit a bruit.

General factors

Do not forget to look for other general signs of hypo- or hyperfunction.

- Myxoedema
  - bradycardia
  - subnormal temperature
  - supraclavicular fat pads
  - rough dry skin
  - slow delayed reflexes
- Thyrotoxicosis
  - tachycardia (even atrial fibrillation)
  - hot sweating hands
  - fine tremor
  - pretibial myxoedema.

Eye signs in thyroid disease

Exophthalmos (Fig. 7.11)

Assess by standing behind the patient and tilting head backwards. Examine the protrusion of the eyeball in relation to the superciliary ridges.

- Mild
  - widening of palpebral fissure due to lid retraction (Stellwag's sign)
  - lid lag may also be present
- Moderate
  - actual bulging due to orbital deposition of fat
  - absence of wrinkling of forehead when patient looks up (Joffroy's sign)
- Severe
  - intraorbital oedema with congestion, raised intraocular pressure and muscle paresis resulting in diplopia (ophthalmoplegia)

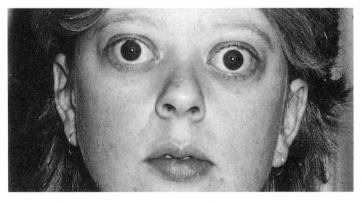

Fig. 7.11 Exophthalmos secondary to Graves'.

— Subsequently there may be difficulty in convergence (Moebius's sign)
- Progressive
  — increases in spite of successful treatment of thyrotoxicosis. Can result in impaired visual acuity due to chemosis, impaired corneal sensitivity and ophthalmoplegia

Causes of exophthalmos
- Endocrine
  — thyrotoxicosis
  — Cushing's syndrome (rare)
  — acromegaly (rare)
- Non-endocrine
  — skull deformity (e.g. craniostenosis)
  — orbital tumours, primary
    — meningioma
    — optic nerve glioma
    — lymphoma
    — osteoma
    — haemangioma
  — orbital tumours, secondary
    — carcinoma of antrum
    — neuroblastoma
    — blood-spread metastases
  — inflammation (e.g. orbital cellulitis)
  — vascular lesions
    — cavernous sinus thrombosis
    — cavernous sinus A-V fistula
    — ophthalmic artery aneurysm
  — eye disease (usually bilateral)
    — severe glaucoma
    — severe myopia.

The breast

History

- Menarche
- Menopause
- Pregnancies
- The pill
- Lactation

- Family history
- Symptom changes during menstrual cycle
- Nipple discharge.

Inspection

- Examine the patient, who should be stripped to the waist, in a semi-recumbent position
- Ask her where the trouble is, as this will help focus attention when looking for minor degrees of skin dimpling or irregularity of breast outline
- Inspect the breast with the patient
  — lying back
  — sitting up
  — with her arms raised
- Look at the size and shape. Is it:
  — regular and symmetrical (Fig. 7.12)
  — distorted
  — larger or smaller than its opposite number?
- Look at the skin.
  — Is it:
    — reddened or discoloured
    — dimpled (Fig. 7.13)

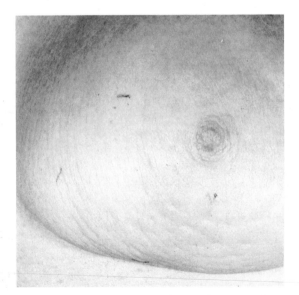

Fig. 7.12 Loss of normal contour of breast due to a carcinoma.

— howing peau d'orange (Fig. 7.14)
— ulcerated (Fig. 7.15)
— scarred?
— Are there any:
— nodules
— dilated veins?

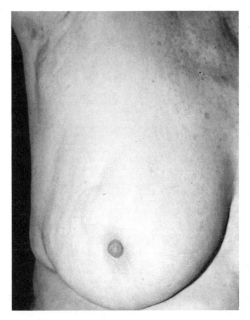

Fig. 7.13 Skin dimpling from a carcinoma of the breast made more marked by elevation of the arms.

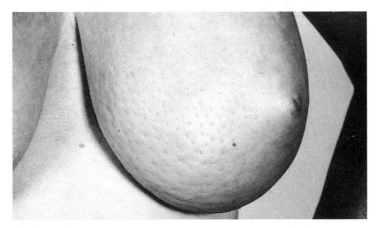

Fig. 7.14 Peau d'orange.

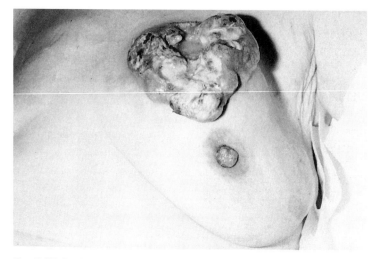

Fig. 7.15 An ulcerating breast cancer.

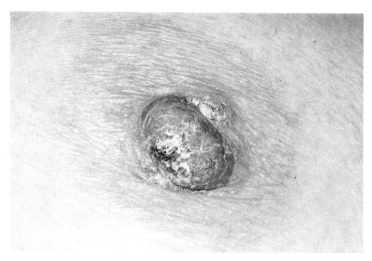

Fig. 7.16 Paget's disease of the nipple.

- Look at the nipple and areola.
  — Is it:
    — retracted
    — cracked
    — ezcematous (e.g. Paget's disease) (Fig. 7.16)
    — over-pigmented?

— Is there any evidence of:
  — retention cysts
  — abscesses
  — mammary fistula or sinus
  — discharge, clear or bloodstained?
- Summary of nipple changes
  — displaced
  — destroyed
  — depressed
  — discoloured
  — duplicated
  — discharging
    — blood
    — serum
    — pus
    — milk.

Palpation

- Start by examining the normal breast, but warn the patient that that is what you are going to do, or else they will think you have made a mistake. This enables you to gauge the normal nodularity and consistency of the individual patient's breast tissue. However, always be on the look-out for bilateral disease.
- Systematically examine all four quadrants of the breast and the axillary tail, both with the flat of the hand and between the pulps of the fingers.
- Palpate behind the nipple, and simultaneously note whether any discharge can be expressed. This may be difficult in the examination if the patient is examined by many candidates.
- Note the consistency of the breast. Is it:
  — soft
  — regular
  — nodular
  — tender?
- If there is a discrete lump, note its:
  — site (in which quadrant)
  — size (in cm)
  — shape
  — consistency
    — hard
    — soft
    — cystic

— overlying skin
   — dimpled
   — ulcerated
   — peau d'orange
— fixity
   — to skin
   — to deep tissue

- If a lump feels cystic, test for fluctuation as described on page 55 (Fig. 7.8)
- Testing for fixation:
   — To skin: gently pinch up skin overlying the lesion.
   — To deep tissue: ask patient to place her hands on her hips. Then pick up the lump gently between your fingers and assess its mobility in two dimensions. Now ask the patient to press in firmly onto her hips and reassess the lump's mobility (Fig. 7.17), again in two dimensions. If the lump is attached deeply to muscle, its mobility will be diminished.

Examination of the axilla

- The patient should be sitting up at an angle of about 60 degrees.
- The left axilla should be examined by the right hand and vice versa.
- Raise the patient's arm with your own non-examining hand, and then pass your examining hand up into the axilla (Fig. 7.18A, B). The patient's arm can now be lowered a little to relax the axillary skin and muscle boundaries. The fingers on the examining hand

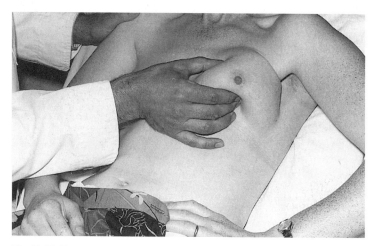

Fig. 7.17 Testing for fixity of a breast lump.

can then probe the axilla for the presence of any enlarged lymph nodes, either in the centre of the axilla, high along the axillary vein or under the pectoralis major muscle. Nodes can often be felt more easily by rolling them over the lateral thoracic wall.

- If nodes are palpable, note their:
  - — size
  - — number
  - — consistency
  - — mobility
  - — fixity

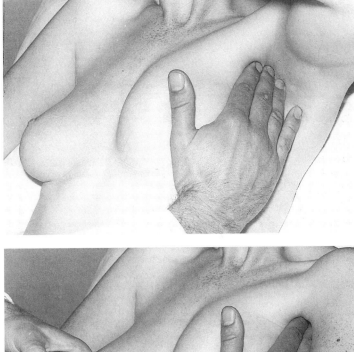

A

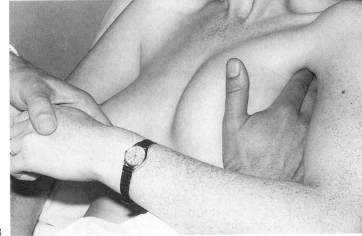

B

Fig. 7.18 Examining the axilla.

- Do not forget to examine both axillae, and also the supraclavicular fossae, as well as the abdomen, chest and the spine if relevant. In the abdomen look for any evidence of hepatomegaly, ascites or masses.
- If faced with a lesion in a male breast (Fig. 7.19), the examination should be almost identical with that of the female breast.

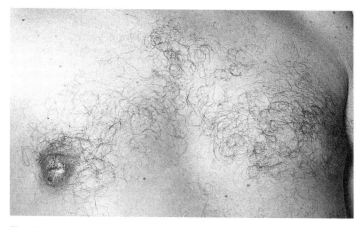

Fig. 7.19 Carcinoma of the male breast.

Clinical bay 2: Musculoskeletal and neurological cases

8

In this bay you may expect to be shown conditions such as:

- Osteoarthritis of hip/knee, etc.
- Rheumatoid arthritis
- Bone tumours
- External fracture fixators
- Carpal tunnnel
- Nerve injuries and entrapment syndromes
- Trigger finger
- Dupuytren's contracture (Fig. 6.6)
- Hallux valgus/rigidus
- Ingrowing toenails
- Ganglia
- Bursae
- Post-traumatic conditions
- Plaster complications

You may also be asked to comment on scans, X-rays and simple procedures such as the reduction of a Colles' fracture.

The orthopaedic examination

Just because the major complaint may appear isolated to bones and joints, do not forget to accurately assess the patient's general health.

Inspection

Skin
- Colour
- Abnormal pattern of skin creases
- Scars
- Sinuses.

Shape

- Deformity
- Swelling
- Oedema
- Wasting
- Lumps
- Shortening — visual assessment
- Position of limb.

Palpation

Skin

- Temperature
- Moisture
- Tenderness
- Sensation
  — light touch
  — pin prick
  — temperature
  — deep pain
  — vibration
  — position sense
- Pulses

Soft tissues

- Oedema
- Soft tissue masses
- Soft tissue tenderness
- Synovial membrane thickening
- Capsular thickening
- Fluid
  — in bursae
  — in joints.

Bones

- Landmarks
- Lumps, single
  — exostoses
  — tumours
    — osteoma
    — chondroma
    — osteoclastoma
    — osteosarcoma, etc.

- Lumps, multiple
  - exostoses (diaphyseal aclasis)
- Tenderness
- Misalignment
- Measure length in cm
  - real
  - apparent (Fig. 8.1A, B).

Movement

Range
- Assess any limitation in all directions, e.g. for the hip
  - flexion
  - extension
  - adduction
  - abduction
  - medial rotation
  - lateral rotation
- Passive movements
- Active movements

A

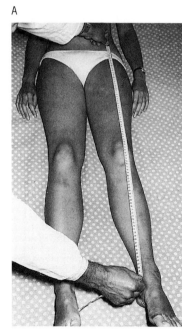

B

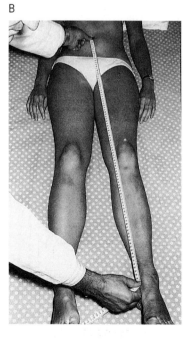

Fig. 8.1 Measuring leg length.
A. Real length — from the anterior superior iliac spine to the medial malleolus.
B. Apparent length — from the umbilicus to the medial malleolus.

- Painful movements
- Abnormal movements.

Muscles
- Power of movement (see p. 76)
- Comparison of sides
- Shape during contraction
- Reflexes.

Function
- Standing
- Lifting
- Control of movements
- Gait.

Causes of joint deformity

Skin
- Contractures, e.g. burns.

Fascia
- Contractures, e.g. Dupuytren's contracture (Fig. 6.6).

Muscle
- Paralysis, e.g. poliomyelitis
- Fibrosis, e.g. Volkmann's ischaemic contracture
- Spasm, e.g. chronic joint inflammation.

Tendon
- Division
- Adhesions.

Ligaments
- Rupture, e.g. rheumatoid arthritis
- Stretching and laxity.

Capsule
- Rupture
- Fibrosis, e.g. osteoarthritis.

Bone
- Malignment, e.g. dislocation, subluxation
- Alteration in shape, e.g. old rickets
- Previous trauma, e.g. malunion
- Pressure atrophy.

Nerves
- neuropathic joints (Fig. 8.2), e.g.:
  — diabetic neuropathy
  — tabes dorsalis
  — syringomyelia
  — leprosy
  — cauda equina lesions.

Peripheral nerves

General comments

Patients with peripheral nerve lesions are easily transportable and often appear in the examination.
- Inspect the limb carefully for:
  — recent scars
  — old wounds
  — deformity suggesting previous fractures
  — any skin changes
  — the state of the nails and hair
  — any evidence of wasting
  — any evidence of ischaemia

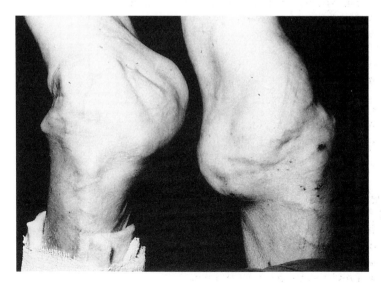

Fig. 8.2 Neuropathic joints (Charcot's).

- Assess motor power
  - Grade 5: normal power
  - Grade 4: contraction against gravity and some resistance
  - Grade 3: contraction against gravity only
  - Grade 2: movement only with gravity eliminated
  - Grade 1: flicker of contraction but no movement
  - Grade 0: complete paralysis
- Assess sensation
  - light touch: use cotton wool
  - pain: use sharp object with great care and record only when sensation is sharp
  - vibration: place vibrating tuning fork over bony prominence
  - temperature: use appropriate stimuli (not practical in the exam).

It is impossible within the confines of this book to give clinical details of all the nerve lesions that may present in the examination. However, a simple approach will be described for the major lesions of the upper limb and this can be applied to lesions elsewhere in the body.

The radial nerve

Causes of injury
- Fractures of the shaft of humerus
- Penetrating wounds to the axilla or arm
- Pressure in the axilla from sitting with the arm suspended over a chair, or over a crutch.

Motor loss
- Axillary or proximal upper arm injury
  - loss of triceps action
  - wrist drop
- Middle third of humerus injury (e.g. fractures)
  - sparing of brachioradialis (when this is paralysed, elbow flexion is weakened)
  - wrist drop
- Posterior interosseous injury
  - wrist drop not present, but hand held in radial deviation when attempting extension
  - unable to maintain finger extension against forcible flexion
- Superficial radial injury
  - no motor loss.

Sensory loss

For all levels of damage to the radial nerve itself, the loss is as depicted in Figure 8.3. However, there is no detectable sensory loss when only the posterior interosseous is injured.

The ulnar nerve

Causes of injury

- Compression at the elbow
- Fracture of the medial epicondyle
- Penetrating injuries at any level
- Delayed palsy with marked cubitus valgus
- Lacerations at the wrist.

Motor loss

- Low lesion at the wrist
  — claw hand with ring and little finger hyperextended at the metacarpophalangeal joint and flexed at the interphalangeal joints
  — wasting of the intrinsic muscles
  — inability to adduct thumb (adductor pollicis paralysis)
  Froment's sign: get patient to grasp paper between thumb and index finger by adducting the thumb. When adductor pollicis is paralysed, the thumb flexes due to contraction of flexor pollicis longus (Fig. 8.4).

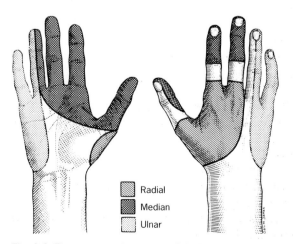

Loss of pin prick sensation with lesions of the major nerves of the upper limb

Radial
Median
Ulnar

Fig. 8.3 The cutaneous innervation of the hand.

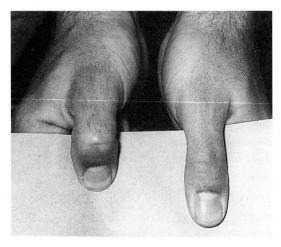

Fig. 8.4 A positive Froment's test on the right hand (i.e. on the left of the illustration).

- High lesion at the elbow
  - claw hand but with terminal interphalangeal joints not flexed as half of flexor profundus is now paralysed
  - wasting of the intrinsic muscles
  - positive Froment's sign
- Very high lesions
  - flexor carpi ulnaris also lost
  - plus same signs as above.

Sensory loss
Lost over the ulnar one-and-a-half fingers (Fig. 8.3).

The median nerve

Causes of injury
- Penetrating injuries
- Lacerations at the wrist: dislocation of the carpal lunate
- Carpal tunnel compression

Motor loss
- Low lesions
  - wasting of the thenar eminence
  - inability to abduct thumb
  - true opposition lost

- Lesions at or above the cubital fossa
  - wasting of the forearm and thenar eminence
  - loss of flexors to thumb and index finger
  - hand often held in benediction position with ulnar fingers flexed and index finger straight.

Sensory loss
- Sensation is lost over the radial three-and-a-half digits (Fig. 8.3). Patient is unable to pick up pin between thumb and index finger.
- Trophic changes are common.

Rapid assessment of upper limb peripheral nerve injury

Three simple clinical findings will help rapid assessment of these nerve lesions:

1. Wrist drop — a radial nerve lesion is present.
2. Positive Froment's sign — an ulnar nerve lesion is present.
3. Loss of ability to flex the index finger — a median nerve lesion is present.

Causes of claw hand

- Ulnar and median nerve palsy
- Volkmann's contracture
- Rheumatoid arthritis
- Brachial plexus lesions
- Spinal cord lesions — syringomyelia
- Poliomyelitis
- Amyotrophic lateral sclerosis.

Clinical bay 3: Circulatory and lymphatic cases

9

In this bay you may expect to see vascular cases including the following:

- Chronic ischaemia of limbs
- Acute ischaemia
- Amputations
- Aneurysms
- Carotid artery disease/TIAs
- A-V fistula (traumatic, idiopathic, iatrogenic)
- Diabetic feet
- Venous disease
  — varicose veins
  — deep vein insufficiency
  — post-phlebitic leg
  — stasis ulcers
- Lymphoedema (Fig. 9.1)
- Hyperhidrosis.

You may also be asked to comment on arteriograms, venograms, duplex scans, Doppler studies.

The vascular case

History

- Age, sex, occupation
- Smoking habits
- Onset of symptoms — acute or chronic
- Pain
  — intermittent claudication:
    — site
    — claudication distance

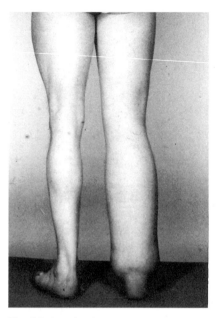

Fig. 9.1 Lymphoedema.

  — onset and progression
  — influence on occupation
 — Rest pain:
   — site
   — sleeping pattern
   — hangs foot out of bed
   — paraesthesia
   — distribution
   — timing.

Past medical history

- Associated diseases:
  — diabetes mellitus
  — scleroderma
  — Buerger's disease
- Associated symptoms:
  — chest pain
  — fainting
  — shortness of breath
  — transient ischaemic attacks

- Previous:
  - — myocardial infarction
  - — stroke
  - — vascular operations
- Drugs:
  - — β-blockers
  - — ergot
  - — anticoagulants.

Examination

The whole of the cardiovascular system should be examined with care, with particular reference to:
- Blood pressure
- Heart
  - — murmurs
  - — rhythm
- Lung fields
  - — crepitations
  - — rhonchi
  - — effusions
- Vascular bruits
  - — aortic
  - — carotid.

The patient's general health is an essential part of the overall assessment of any vascular case.

Inspection

- With leg
  - — horizontal
  - — elevated
  - — dependent
- Colour
  - — marble-white
  - — waxy pallor
  - — cyanosed
  - — mottled
  - — ischaemic rubor
  - — haemosiderin deposits
- Trophic changes
  - — thickening and scaling of skin
  - — wasting of toes or finger pulps

— blistering
— loss of hair (unreliable)
- Oedema
- Distended or guttered veins
- Pressure areas: check the
  — heel
  — malleoli
  — tips of toes
  — between toes
  — head of fifth metatarsal
  — ball of foot
- Ulceration
  — ischaemic
  — pressure sores
  — venous stasis
- Gangrenous digits (Fig. 9.2)
- Scars
  — old injury
  — previous vascular surgery
  — check abdomen for old sympathectomy scar
- Amputations

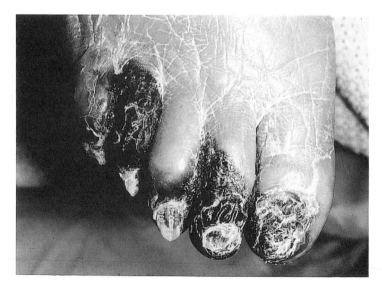

Fig. 9.2 Gangrenous digits.

Palpation

- Temperature: compare limbs
- Capillary return: press toe pulp until blanched and then observe time for area to turn pink again
- Pulses
  — femoral: below inguinal ligament at midpoint between anterior superior iliac spine and symphysis pubis
  — popliteal: flex knee to a right angle and palpate deeply with fingers of both hands against the posterior surface of the upper tibia (Fig. 9.3)
  — dorsalis pedis: runs from midpoint between the malleoli to the cleft between first and second metatarsal, usually just lateral to extensor hallucis longus
  — posterior tibial: halfway between back of medial malleolus and medial border of tendon Achilles
- Measure pulse pressures wherever possible. If normal foot pulses are absent, they may be replaced occasionally by the peroneal artery. If the patient describes intermittent claudication and yet still has peripheral pulses, then exercise the patient and the pulses may disappear.
- Do not forget to examine the carotid, subclavian, brachial, radial and ulnar pulses as well.

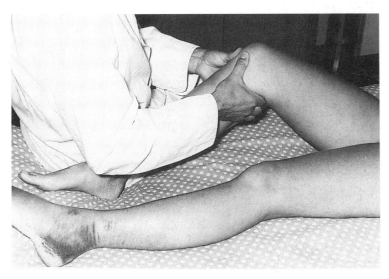

Fig. 9.3 Examining the popliteal artery.

Buerger's vascular angle

Elevate the limb and measure the angle at which the limb develops a cadaveric pallor with guttering of the veins. A normal limb can be raised to 90 degrees and still remain pink, while a vascular angle of less than 20 degrees indicates severe ischaemia. The height in centimetres between sternum and heel when the foot blanches is approximately equal to the pressure in foot vessels in millimetres of mercury.

Capillary filling time

After elevating the limb, then rest it dependently and an ischaemic limb will turn from white to a ruddy dusky cyanosed hue. A normal limb will remain a healthy pink colour. The time taken for the foot to become pink is the capillary filling time and may be up to 20 seconds in an ischaemic foot.

Venous assessment

Look for signs of deep vein thrombosis:

- Oedema
- Distended veins
- Increased temperature
- Increased girth
- Calf tenderness
- Homan's sign — pain or dorsiflexing the foot with the knee extended

Auscultation

Listen for bruits over all major arteries:

- Carotids
- Brachials
- Aorta
- Renals
- Femorals

Don't forget to compare sides and limbs for pulse status, blood pressure and bruits.

Varicose veins

Inspection

- Stand the patient up

- Carefully examine both legs from lower abdomen to toes, both front and back
- Assess anatomical distribution of the veins
- Look for a saphena varix
- Look for any evidence of varicose eczema, lipodermatosclerosis or ulceration. Varicose ulcers are:
  — shallow
  — irregular
  — usually surrounded by:
    — fine venules (venous flare)
    — pigmentation (haemosiderin)
    — eczematous scaly skin
  — usually sited just above the medial malleolus
- Look for any scars that might suggest previous surgical treatment
- Look for any evidence of oedema or swelling that might indicate deep vein involvement
- Do not forget to examine the lower abdomen and pubes adequately.

Palpation

- Gently palpate the veins.
- Is there a cough impulse? There may be a fluid thrill over the saphenous opening. This is particularly marked when there is a saphena varix present (Cruveilhier's sign).
- Chevrier's tap sign: with the patient still standing, tap the distal varicosities and this will impart an impulse or fluid thrill to a finger placed proximally just below the saphenous opening.
- Brodie–Trendelenberg test (Fig. 9.4A, B, C): lie the patient down and elevate the limb to empty the veins of blood. Then apply a high tourniquet or press over the saphenous opening and stand the patient up again. If the veins remain empty, this suggests that the incompetence is at the saphenofemoral junction. This can be confirmed by removing the pressure and observing that the veins immediately fill again. If, however, the veins fill again despite pressure being applied at the saphenous opening, this implies that there are communicating perforators lower down in the limb. Using a tourniquet, pressure should be applied further down the limb until, after standing, the veins are controlled. This will indicate the level of the perforators.
- Morrissey's test for saphenofemoral incompetence: empty the veins by elevating the leg to about 30 degrees, and then get the patient to cough. Incompetence is confirmed if retrograde filling of the veins is seen.

- Fegan's method for localizing perforators: mark the veins with the patient standing, and then elevate the limb. Palpation down the course of the vein may then reveal defects in the deep fascia which will represent the sites of perforating veins.
- Test for deep vein patency: place a tourniquet around the thigh and get the patient to walk for about five minutes. If the deep veins are occluded, the patient will experience a severe bursting pain in the leg (this test is virtually impossible in the examination, as time is at a premium, but it is vital to know how to test for deep vein patency in case you are asked to describe how it is done).

Auscultation

- This is rarely necessary, but in certain severe cases a venous hum may be heard over a saphena varix
- If there is an arteriovenous fistula causing the varicosities, a loud bruit may be heard.

A   B   C

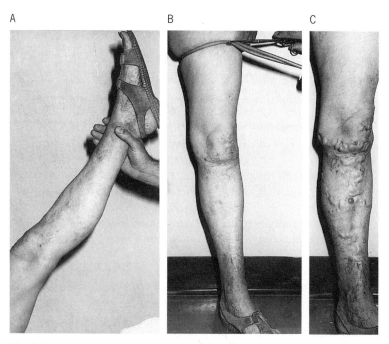

Fig. 9.4 The Brodie–Trendelenberg test.
A. Elevate the limb to empty the veins.
B. Apply a high tourniquet and then stand the patient up – the veins will be controlled and not fill if the incompetence is above the tourniquet site.
C. The veins will fill after releasing the tourniquet.

General comments

With all cases of varicose veins it is vital to assess the patient carefully and to decide whether the varicosities are primary or secondary.

Secondary varicose veins can be caused by:

- Deep vein thrombosis
- Pregnancy
- Intrapelvic neoplasia (cervix, ovary, rectum)
- Arteriovenous fistula.

Clinical bay 4: The abdomen and trunk

10

In this bay you may expect to see the following types of cases:

- Abdominal masses
  - spleen
  - liver
  - kidney
  - gall bladder
  - tumours of the stomach, bowel, etc.
  - pancreatic masses
  - ovarian masses
- Liver disease
  - cirrhosis
  - jaundice
  - ascites
  - lymphoma
  - tumours
    - primary
    - metastatic
- Stomas
- Herniae
  - inguinal
  - femoral
  - umbilical
  - incisional
  - elsewhere
- Scrotal masses
  - tumours
  - inflammatory swellings
  - hydroceles
  - epididymal cysts
- Immunosuppressed patients
  - renal transplants

— opportunistic infections
— Kaposi's sarcoma
● Appliances
— prostheses (e.g. breast)
— trusses
— corsets.

You may also be asked to comment upon relevant investigations, such as ultrasound, CT and MRI scans, barium studies, abdominal arteriograms, renal imaging, blood results, etc.

The abdomen

Inspection

Position the patient carefully, with the patient's head resting on a pillow to relax the recti. Expose the complete abdomen which will remind you to examine the hernial orifices and genitalia. Keyhole examination is not acceptable.

Look at the abdomen's:

● Size
● Shape
● Symmetry
● Movement with respiration

Look for:

● Scars
● Distension
— flatus
— faeces
— foetus
— fat
— fluid
— ascites
— encysted
— fibroids or other large masses
— hepatomegaly
— splenomegaly
— polycystic kidneys
— retroperitoneal tumours
● Visible peristalsis

- Discoloration
  — Cullen's sign (periumbilical)
  — Grey Turner's sign (flanks)
  — erythema ab igne (guide to localization of pain) (Fig. 10.1)
- Rashes
- Bruising
- Excoriation
- Dilated veins
  — caput medusae — blood flows away from umbilicus
  — inferior vena cava obstruction — blood flows in a cephalic direction
- Lumps
- Herniae
- Sinuses or fistulae.

Palpation

This must be done methodically.

1. *Light* palpation should be undertaken first, looking for tenderness. Watch the patient's face. *Do not hurt the patient.*
2. *Deep* palpation should then be undertaken looking for deep tenderness and abdominal masses.

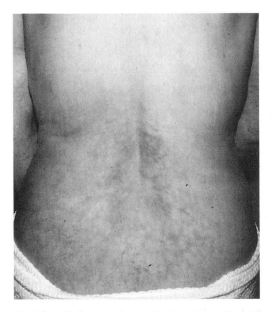

Fig. 10.1 Erythema ab igne on the back in a patient with carcinoma of the pancreas.

3. Do not forget to examine the:
   - Supraclavicular fossae
   - Hernial orifices
   - Genitalia
   - Femoral pulses.

(Rectal and vaginal examinations are not allowed.)

Abdominal masses

Describe any abdominal mass by eliciting the following signs:

- Position
- Size
- Shape — regular or irregular
- Edge — distinct or indistinct
- Consistency — solid or cystic
- Pulsatile or transmitted pulsation
- Mobile or fixed
- Does it move on respiration?
- Tympanitic or dull to percussion
- Associated with abnormal bowel sounds or bruits.

(Never express an opinion on a pelvic mass until assured that the bladder is empty.)

Liver *(Fig. 10.2)*
- Right hypochondrial mass
- Cannot get above it
- Moves down on respiration
- Dull to percussion.

Spleen *(Fig. 10.3)*
- Left hypochondrial mass
- Moves down and medially towards umbilicus on respiration
- Sharp anterior edge directed downwards and inwards and may be notched
- Unable to get above it, but with a space posteriorly between the organ and sacrospinalis
- Dull to percussion.

Kidney *(Fig. 10.4)*
- Loin mass
- Bimanually palpable
- May be ballotable

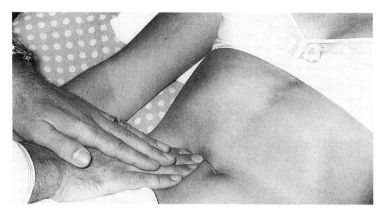

Fig. 10.2 Examining the liver.

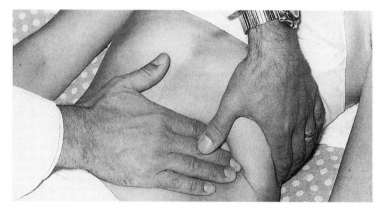

Fig. 10.3 Examining the spleen.

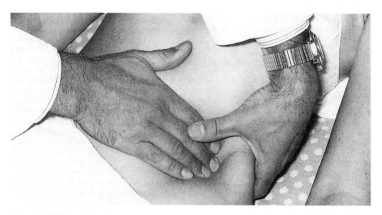

Fig. 10.4 Examining the kidney.

- Moves down on respiration
- Dull to percussion but often with a band of colonic resonance anteriorly.

Percussion

- Dull or resonant over any masses
- Dull to percussion over a full bladder (this will usually signify chronic retention as acute retention is not likely to appear in the examination and is painful)
- Test for shifting dullness associated with ascites.

Auscultation

- Bowel sounds — borborygmi:
  - silent: paralytic ileus or secondary to abdominal catastrophe (unlikely in the examination)
  - normal
  - hyperactive borborygmi (associated with obstruction)
  - high-pitched or tinkling sounds (associated with bowel distension due to obstruction)
- Bruits: listen over aorta, iliac arteries and renal arteries
- Succussion splash: a sign of pyloric stenosis.

The groin and scrotum

Inspection

- During examination of the groin and scrotum, always remember to compare clinical findings with the opposite side. For example, a large right inguinal hernia may be accompanied by a very prominent cough impulse or smaller hernia on the left
- Look with the patient lying down, and then stand him up
- Look for:
  - any swelling, especially when the patient is asked to cough
  - any scars
  - any sinuses
  - the position and lie of the testes, e.g. the testis hangs low with a varicocele (Fig. 10.5), while a horizontal position is associated with torsion (Fig. 10.6)
  - discoloration, e.g.:
    - saphena varix
    - strangled hernia (this is not likely to appear in the exam)

— oedema
  — idiopathic
  — cardiac
  — infective
— ulceration
  — idiopathic scrotal gangrene (Fournier's gangrene — again
    unlikely to appear in the exam)
  — carcinoma
— nodules, e.g. sebaceous cysts of the scrotum
— Malgaigne's bulges — seen in thin individuals with poor
  musculature.

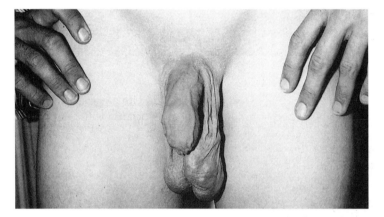

Fig. 10.5 A varicocele.

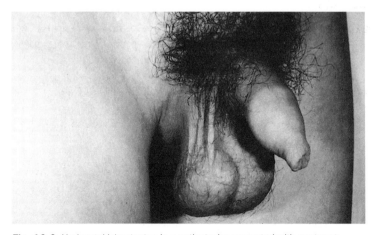

Fig. 10.6 Horizontal lying testes in a patient who presented with recurrent
attacks of torsion.

Palpation

Is there a palpable impulse? Assess with the patient standing, and use the appropriate hand for each side, i.e. the right hand for the right side, etc. Place the index finger over the deep ring, the middle finger over Hesselbach's triangle, and the ring finger over the femoral canal. Then ask the patient to turn his head to the opposite side and give a cough.

Hesselbach's triangle is bounded by:
1. The inferior epigastric artery
2. The inguinal ligament
3. The lateral border of rectus abdominis.

- Is there a swelling?
- If there is, can you get above it?
  — yes: then the swelling is not issuing from the inguinal canal
  — no: then the swelling may be issuing from the inguinal canal
- Is it:
  — tender
  — reducible
  — fluctuant
  — mobile
  — pulsatile
  — translucent?
- What is its anatomical position in relation to the:
  — pubic tubercle
  — femoral canal
  — femoral vessels
  — neck of the scrotum?
- Are there any other associated abnormalities? e.g.:
  — hydrocele associated with an inguinal hernia in children
  — leg or perineal sepsis associated with groin lymphadenopathy
  — varicose veins associated with a saphena varix?

Auscultation

- Do not forget to listen to swellings in the groin
- A large inguinal hernia containing bowel may well exhibit bowel sounds
- A femoral aneurysm or arteriovenous fistula will usually have a bruit.

Transillumination

- This can be a very valuable physical sign
- Hydroceles of the cord will possess the same brilliant translucency as scrotal hydroceles or epidydimal cysts.

Herniae

- Is it reducible?

Lie the patient down — it may reduce itself. If not, then gently apply pressure around the neck and squeeze the fundus, again extremely gently. This procedure is termed *taxis*.

Taxis should not be applied when:

1. There is accompanying intestinal obstruction.
2. There are any signs of strangulation, e.g. tenderness, redness or skin discoloration, oedema of the skin.
3. When a hernia has been irreducible for weeks.

- What are its contents?
  - bowel: difficult to reduce initially, while the last part goes easily with a gurgle
  - omentum: feels doughy, and reduces easily initially, but the last part is difficult due to adhesions to the sac
- What is its relation to the:
  - pubic tubercle (in fat patients in whom this landmark is difficult to find, follow up the tendon of abductor longus to its bony insertion)
  - femoral canal
  - Hesselbach's triangle?

Indirect inguinal hernia

- Exhibits cough impulse at superficial ring. Some surgeons advocate invaginating the little finger up through the scrotum to the superficial ring — but this is painful and unnecessary
- If reducible, can be controlled by pressure over the deep ring (just above the halfway point between the symphysis pubis and the anterior superior iliac spine)
- The sac will lie above and medial to the pubic tubercle
- May protrude down into the scrotum or labia
- Three forms are described:
  - bubonocele: confined to the inguinal canal
  - funicular: protruding into the scrotum, but separate from the testis
  - complete: patent processus vaginalis, with testis appearing to lie within distal sac
- Once reduced, the bulge reappears at mid-inguinal point.

Direct inguinal hernia

- Bulges through Hesselbach's triangle
- Not controlled by pressure over the deep ring
- Reduces almost immediately on lying the patient down
- Once reduced, the bulge reappears exactly where it was reduced, i.e. just above and medial to pubic tubercle.

Femoral hernia

- The inguinal canal is empty with no cough impulse at the superficial ring
- The neck is below and lateral to the pubic tubercle
- Because of the blending of the fascia, the downward extension of the sac is prevented, and the sac may mount up over the inguinal ligament. However, the neck will still be below and lateral to the pubic tubercle
- Irreducibility is ten times more common in femoral herniae than in inguinal herniae.

Differential diagnoses (Fig. 10.7)

- Scrotal swellings — you can get above them
- Hydrocele of the cord — localized, moves with traction on the testis and can be transilluminated
- Undescended testis — the scrotum is empty, and can also be associated with an accompanying indirect inguinal hernia
- Lipoma of the cord — soft, non-tender with no cough impulse. Can also be associated with an inguinal hernia
- Saphena varix — softer than a femoral hernia, blue, non-tender, associated with varicosities of the long saphenous vein with a positive Cruveilhier's sign (a marked fluid thrill on coughing)
- Lymph node — especially difficult to differentiate from a strangulated femoral hernia. Look for focus of infection in the feet or perineum
- Psoas abscess — swelling lateral to the femoral artery often with evidence of back or intra-abdominal disease
- Femoral aneurysm — expansile, pulsatile swelling often with a bruit.

The scrotum

- Are there any skin abnormalities?
  — wounds
  — ulcers

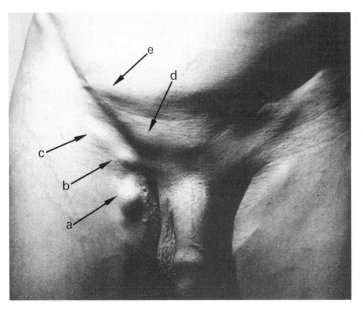

Fig. 10.7 Multiple groin swellings.
a. Saphena varix.   b. Femoral hernia.   c. Femoral artery aneurysm.
d. Inguinal hernia.   e. Inguinal lymph node.

— sinuses
— tumour
- Are both testes satisfactorily in the scrotum?
- Examine and compare both testes. Are they normal in respect of:
  — lie
  — size
  — consistency
- Examine the epididymis (body, globus major, globus minor)
- Palpate the cord, feeling for the vas
- Are there any masses? (You can get above any scrotal mass)
- Is the mass solid or cystic?
  1. Solid
     — is it confined to the testis?
       — non-tender
         — neoplasm (Fig. 10.8)
         — old clotted haematocele
         — syphilitic gumma (very rare now)
       — tender
         — chronic torsion
         — severe orchitis

— is it confined to the epididymis?
- epididymitis
- acute: red, hot, enlarged, tender
- chronic: tuberculosis
2. Cystic
- assess the position of the testis by means of palpation and transillumination
- is the testis within the cystic swelling?
- vaginal hydrocele
- is the testis separate from the cystic swelling
- epididymal cyst
- spermatocele
- is there a small cyst at the upper pole — cyst of hydatid of Morgagni
- Beware: a secondary hydrocele may mask underlying disease of the testis
- Vascular: are the veins of the pampiniform plexus dilated and varicose? — a varicocele (Fig. 10.5)
- When examining the scrotum and groins, do not omit examination of the penis. Exclude:
  - phimosis
  - hypospadias
  - balanitis
  - carcinoma, etc.

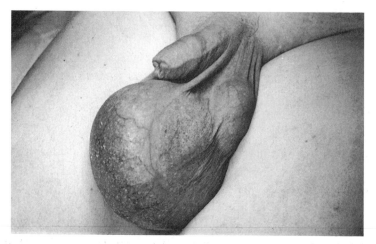

Fig. 10.8 Testicular tumour.

Clinical bay 5: Communication skills and general guidelines 11

Communication skills

In this bay you may well encounter actors who will have been previously briefed to act out a certain clinical situation or vignette. This section is not a test of knowledge but is designed to assess a candidate's ability to communicate effectively with patients, relatives or colleagues. Each vignette will be designed to allow the examiners to observe the candidate's ability to cope with the situation and effectively to communicate such matters as are relevant to the individual concerned. It is difficult to prepare specifically for this section of the examination other than to spend time clinically in hospital practice in which such situational circumstances arise. The types of 'clinical situations' which may be presented could well include:

- Obtaining informed consent for a particular operative procedure, e.g.:
  — thyroidectomy
  — aortic aneurysm
  — low anterior resection
  — laparoscopic cholecystectomy
- Obtaining consent for a post-mortem from relatives
- Discussing a complaint with a patient or relative
- Discussing diagnosis and treatment of a difficult condition
- Discussing a poor prognosis with a patient or relative
- Discussion with relatives after the death of a family member
- Talking to a dying patient
- Discussing a patient's possible entry into a research trial
- Discussing operative risks with a patient who refuses blood transfusions.

For each of the above scenarios it may help you in your preparation to prepare lists of general principles or facts that you would need to cover, e.g.

- Introduce yourself
- Ensure that patient or relative is sitting in a comfortable manner and environment
- Review of facts as understood by patient or relative
- Explanation as necessary
- Specific explanations dependent on scenario or clinical procedure
- Prognosis whenever applicable
- Apology whenever applicable
- Condolescences whenever applicable
- Agree action plan
- Check understanding
- Always finish with question as to whether there is any other matter that the patient or relative would wish to ask you or to discuss.

Never ever lose your temper or demonstrate your frustration.

The options are limitless but all scenarios will have a strong clinical bias and will represent possible real-life situations. It is important to keep a clear head in this part of the examination, not to panic or clam up, and above all to *'think clinical'*.

General guidelines

During the clinical part of the examination remember:

- That the cases are usually easily transportable, are not acutely ill, and are the type of patient that you are likely to meet day by day in the outpatient department. The candidates who do well in the clinical part of the examination are those who have acquired considerable clinical experience on the wards and in outpatients. Take every opportunity you can of examining physical signs, as it helps substantially if you have encountered the lesion before being confronted by it in the examination itself. Furthermore, take every opportunity not only to communicate with patients and relatives yourself but also watch experienced clinicians handle difficult situations.
- That once you have presented a detailed history and examination, you may not always be in a position to give a definite diagnosis. Don't panic in this situation but try to suggest a working diagnosis or differential diagnoses. It is far more important to be able to give a reasoned opinion and present a practical plan of management. Therefore, while taking the history and making the examination,

it is wise to consider these aspects of the case and come to definite conclusions about them, being prepared to discuss the reasons for your conclusions.

- That it is advisable to wash your hands if possible after visiting a case. This indicates a practical approach to clinical work, and suggests that the candidate has acquired this habit in the ward, even if his or her seniors and betters may tend to ignore it. However, in this and other matters, do not insist if it becomes obvious that it would not be practical in the examination setting.
- That it is not good manners to address the examiner with your legs crossed or with your hands in your pockets.
- Not to talk too fast, and remember to speak up without being too loud. Be very careful to say nothing in the patient's hearing which might be hurtful or alarming. It is usual for the examiner to discuss the case away from the patient, but the examiner may take you back to examine the patient in order to elicit certain physical signs.

For further hints on examination technique, see Chapter 16.

Three golden rules

1. Examine the patient.
2. Do not jump to conclusions.
3. Be thorough.

The viva voce examination

12

General comments

As described in Chapter 3, there are three vivas in this section and these will last a total of 1 hour. Each viva will last for 20 minutes and consist of two 10-minute vivas from a pair of examiners.

The three vivas will be of similar content for all colleges, although they may vary slightly in order and emphasis. For example, the English College vivas comprise:

- Applied surgical anatomy with operative surgery
- Applied physiology and critical care
- Clinical pathology with principles of surgery,

while the Edinburgh College vivas comprise:

- Critical care
- Principles of surgery including operative surgery and applied anatomy
- Clinical surgery and pathology based on the experience demonstrated in the candidate's log book.

For each viva there will be a pair of examiners, who will take turns to ask questions for 10 minutes each. For the English College Operative Surgery oral there will be three examiners, to allow one to examine the log book during the viva. It is essential that log books are brought to this section of the examination.

Before sitting the viva voce section of the examination, candidates must have been awarded a 'pass' in both MCQ papers and the clinical section, as well as having satisfactorily completed the Intercollegiate Basic Surgical Skills course.

For further administrative requirements and regulations see Chapters 1 and 3.

Viva technique

The questions in the viva voce section will tend to cover the whole syllabus, but individual subjects will be considered within the appropriate viva — e.g. questions on the principles of appendicectomy will be asked within the Operative Surgery viva, while pain relief may well be asked in the Critical Care viva.

The examiners will be unlikely to ask you questions that merely elicit specific factual knowledge, as this will have been tested by the MCQ papers. They are more likely to raise topics for discussion in order to assess a candidate's ability to apply knowledge. It is impossible to give any specific advice as to how to prepare for this part of the examination other than to encourage candidates to 'think clinical' and get colleagues to viva them wherever and whenever possible.

It is wise to be aware of any current topics of interest within the sphere of surgery, such as any new therapeutic advances, new aetiological theories, or new approaches in the management of common clinical conditions. This will give the impression of a candidate who is abreast of current surgical thinking and cannot fail but to impress.

Seek to formulate your answer as much as possible. It shows maturity of understanding if you present your answer in a logical progression, and therefore some prepared classifications are useful, e.g.:

- Classification of a clinical condition
  (e.g. intestinal obstruction)
- Classification of treatment modalities
  (e.g. haemorrhoids)
- Classification of surgical complications
  (e.g. post-gastric surgery).

These three examples will be described in detail, merely to illustrate what can be applied to other conditions, therapies, complications, etc.

Classification of intestinal obstruction

1. Functional
   - Paralytic, e.g. postoperative ileus, colonic pseudo-obstruction
   - Mechanical, e.g. strangulated hernia, carcinoma of the colon.

2. Speed of onset
   - Acute, e.g. strangulated hernia
   - Acute-on-chronic, e.g. adhesional obstruction
   - Chronic, e.g. inflammatory fibrous stricture, Crohn's disease.

3. Site
   - Very high, e.g. pyloric stenosis
   - High small bowel, e.g. jejunal tumour
   - Distal small bowel, e.g. gallstone ileus
   - Low colon, e.g. sigmoid carcinoma.

4. Nature
   - Simple, e.g. carcinoma of the colon
   - Strangulated, e.g. strangulated hernia.

5. Aetiology
   - In the lumen, e.g. gallstone ileus
   - In the wall, e.g. carcinoma
   - Outside the wall, e.g. band obstruction, hernia.

Classification of treatment options

1. Prevention
   - Screening programmes
   - Epidemiological factors
   - Prophylaxis.

2. Conservative management
   - Dietary, e.g. high fibre, low fat
   - Medication
     — general, e.g. iron for anaemia
     — specific, e.g. triple therapy for *Helicobacter*
     — prophylactic, e.g. vitamin B_{12} after gastrectomy
     — adjuvant, e.g. chemotherapy with surgery for breast cancer.
   - Mechanical
     — truss for hernias
     — corset for spinal problems
     — walking aids for orthopaedic or vascular cases
     — prostheses for amputees, etc.
   - Rehabilitation
     — physiotherapy
     — occupational therapy
     — altering lifestyle, home facilities, etc.

- MICLO: do *not* forget <u>M</u>asterly <u>I</u>nactivity and <u>C</u>at-<u>L</u>ike <u>O</u>bservation

3. Surgical management
   - Prophylactic, e.g. prophylactic appendicectomy. In the author's view, *not* to be encouraged
   - Curative: hopefully the majority of procedures
   - Palliative, e.g. colonic resection of neoplasia in spite of hepatic metastases in order to prevent obstruction, bleeding, perforation, etc.

This outline may be illustrated in practice with reference to:

The treatment of haemorrhoids

1. Prevention
   - Educate public to avoid constipation
   - High-fibre diet for population.

2. Conservative management
   - Avoid constipation
   - Avoid straining at stool
   - High-fibre diet and bran
   - Appropriate use of laxatives.

3. Surgical management
   - Outpatient procedures
     — phenol injection
     — banding
     — infrared coagulation
   - Day case procedures
     — anal stretch (no longer recommended)
     — cryosurgery (lost a little favour)
     — certain forms of haemorrhoidectomy
   - Inpatient procedures: formal standard haemorrhoidectomy.

Surgical complications

1. Site
   - General
   - Local.

2. Timing
   - Immediate: within 24 hours of surgery
   - Early: within 2–3 weeks of surgery
   - Late: remote from surgery.

This outline may be illustrated in practice with reference to:

The complications following gastric surgery

General
- Immediate
  — inhaled vomit
  — obstructed airway
- Early
  — pulmonary atelectasis
  — bronchopneumonia
  — deep vein thrombosis
  — pulmonary embolism
  — urinary retention
- Late
  — iron deficiency anaemia
  — vitamin B_{12} deficiency
  — steatorrhoea
  — diarrhoea
  — dumping (early and late)
  — osteoporosis
  — reactivated pulmonary tuberculosis.

Local
- Immediate: reactionary haemorrhage
- Early
  — paralytic ileus
  — anastomotic breakdown
  — gastric fistula
  — secondary haemorrhage
  — wound infection
  — wound dehiscence
  — intraperitoneal sepsis
    — peritonitis
    — subphrenic abscess
    — pelvic abscess
  — obstruction due to internal herniation
- Late
  — obstruction due to:
    — adhesions
    — internal herniation
  — afferent loop obstruction
  — small stomach syndrome

— weight loss
— stomal ulcer
— stump carcinoma
— incisional hernia.

It is impossible within the scope of this book to cover adequately all surgically related topics that are likely to come up in the viva voce part of the examination. However, the next three chapters will seek to cover certain practical aspects of clinical surgery that may well be raised within each of the appropriate vivas, and stimulate further reading.

Applied surgical anatomy with operative surgery

13

During this viva you will spend the first 10 minutes talking about relevant surgical anatomy. You may be shown anatomical prosections, bones or X-rays and asked to identify surgical anatomy, such as a cross-section of the abdomen on a CT scan or vessels on an arteriogram. Surgical instruments or equipment will also be available for comment and discussion but there will be *no* histology slides.

There may be live models available for you to demonstrate surface anatomy, surface marking for deeper structures or the siting of certain incisions (see Fig. 13.1)

During this first part of the viva your log book will be examined by one of the surgeon examiners and will undoubtedly form the basis for the subsequent questioning on operative surgery during the second 10 minutes of the viva. It is extremely unlikely that you will be asked any procedure that does not appear within your log book. Therefore it is wise to spend some time going through your own log book and ensure that you feel confident to describe any procedure that appears there.

It helps considerably in this part of the examination if you can include as many practical tips and points of interest as possible, as this will indicate that you have actually performed the asked procedure, or at least assisted at it.

Always remember pre-operative preparation in your description, although some examiners may ask you to omit this and just describe the operation. Therefore be prepared to adapt to the examiner's requests and simply answer the questions put to you.

Do not be surprised if you are asked something very straightforward, such as the removal of a toenail, excision of a sebaceous cyst or appendicectomy. However, be wary, as the examiner will expect you to be able to answer such a straightforward question with great efficiency and accuracy, including such detail as skin preparation, local anaesthetic doses and hazards, etc.

How to describe an operation

Pre-operative preparation

1. Consent: All patients should give informed consent for all procedures.

2. Rehydration: In emergency cases do not forget the need for rehydration by an intravenous infusion to correct any electrolyte disturbance, particularly if the patient has been vomiting.

3. Nasogastric tube: A nasogastric tube (e.g. a 15F oesophageal tube with side holes) is essential pre-operatively if the patient is obstructed, as any vomiting on induction may lead to inhalation problems.

4. Urinary catheter: For any lower abdominal or pelvic surgery, an empty bladder is necessary. A catheter (e.g. a 16F Foley catheter) is also essential for any sick or shocked patient undergoing major surgery in order to monitor their intraoperative urinary output.

5. Crossmatched blood: There is a tendency to over-crossmatch blood for surgery, but certain procedures require that blood should be immediately available, while other procedures merely require that the patient's serum is grouped and saved.

6. Premedication: This is usually left to the anaesthetist to prescribe, but it is wise to be aware of those agents in common current use. No premedication is given in the case of neurosurgery for head injuries, or for any unconscious patient.

7. Starved: If general anaesthesia is employed, patients should be starved for at least 4 hours.

8. Marking: All unilateral lesions or limbs that are to be subjected to surgery should be clearly marked with an indelible pen. Varicose veins are another example where the surgeon himself should mark the lesions pre-operatively with the patient standing up. Stoma siting pre-operatively is strongly recommended.

9. Shaving: This is a debatable point. Most surgeons like to work in a pre-operatively shaved field, although others feel that this is counterproductive and may actually increase the incidence of wound infections.

10. Prophylaxis
    - Antibiotics:
        — There is now strong evidence that antibiotic prophylaxis
        plays a major role in preventing postoperative sepsis.
        This is particularly the case when implants are used,
        e.g. vascular surgery, insertion of orthopaedic prostheses,
        cardiac valve replacements, mammary prostheses, etc.
        — It is also advisable to use such prophylaxis when
        endogenous contamination is high, e.g. gastrointestinal,
        biliary and colorectal surgery.
        — Current policy tends to indicate the use of a broad-
        spectrum cephalosporin in most instances, with the
        addition of an anti-anaerobic agent like metronidazole,
        when the large bowel is involved. Such regimens are
        inevitably tailored to the patient's needs, and should be
        started pre-operatively at induction of anaesthesia
        (see p. 136).
    - Antithrombotic precautions: Most surgeons use these
    routinely, while others tend to reserve them for high-risk
    cases, e.g. elderly, obese, on the pill, previous thrombotic
    episodes, malignancy, polycythaemia, etc. (See p. 138 for
    details of regimens and protocols.)

11. Special requirements
    - Steroids: Patients on long-term steroid therapy are in a state
    of adrenal cortical suppression, and therefore will require
    extra replacement steroids to cover the extra needs of
    surgery: 100–200 mg of hydrocortisone pre-operatively,
    continued postoperatively at a dose regimen dependent on
    the previous steroid dosage.
    - Jaundice
        — A jaundiced patient may well have defective clotting
        abilities and therefore will require vitamin K parenterally
        to correct this (10 mg vitamin K_1 daily, preferably
        intravenously, to minimize the risk of intramuscular
        haematoma formation).
        — An adequate urinary output during induction and
        surgery is necessary, and therefore satisfactory hydration
        during the peri-operative period is essential. Some
        surgeons use a 40–50 g mannitol infusion to induce a
        peri-operative diuresis in an attempt to prevent renal
        failure. A pre-operative infusion of low-dose dopamine
        may protect the kidneys.

- Diabetes: Diabetic patients will require special care in monitoring the glucose level, especially in the emergency situation. Wherever possible diabetic patients should be placed first on the operating list. A possible management protocol may be:

  Diet controlled
  — no specific action required
  — If hyperglycaemia occurs then a sliding scale of insulin should be used, or a glucose-potassium-insulin infusion
  Oral hypoglycaemics
  — omit agents on day of surgery
  — long-acting agents should be stopped the day before surgery (e.g. chlorpropamide)
  — monitor blood glucose in peri- and postoperative period. If hyperglycaemia occurs consider sliding scale or glucose-potassium-insulin infusion
  — resume hypoglycaemic agents on return to full enteral diet
  Insulin dependence
  — omit morning dose of insulin
  — if prompt return to enteral feeding anticipated then consider glucose-potassium-insulin infusion
  — if delayed return to enteral feeding then start sliding scale insulin infusion

  Sliding scale
  — the dose used should be related to the degree of hyperglycaemia. Blood glucose should be monitored regularly and not be allowed to fall below 7 mmol/l
  Glucose-potassium-insulin infusion (Alberti regimen)
  — 16 units of soluble insulin and 10 mmol potassium chloride in 500 ml 10% glucose are infused at 100 ml/hour. The infusion should be started 1 hour before surgery and blood glucose measured after 2 hours. If this is greater than 10 mmol/l then the dose of insulin should be increased by 4 units and the blood glucose rechecked

- Miscellaneous requirements, e.g.:
  — vocal cord check prior to thyroidectomy
  — plain X-ray on the way to theatre to confirm the position of a stone prior to ureterolithotomy.

12. Bowel preparation: Patients' requirements and surgeons' preferences differ greatly. No single regimen will work perfectly on every patient, but it is wise to have a standard preparation to describe, which can also apply to colonoscopy. A typical regimen might be:

- Stop any constipating agents and iron preparations 3–4 days pre-operatively.
- Low-residue diet, and preferably fluid diet for 48 hours prior to surgery.
- Adequate purgation on afternoon prior to surgery, to produce fluid diarrhoea, e.g. magnesium sulphate (2-hourly doses until copious diarrhoea is produced), Klean-prep, Picolax, etc.
- Water, saline or purgative (bisacodyl) enemas administered 1–2 hours pre-operatively until returns are clear.
- Other possible regimens include total gut irrigation with 6–10 litres of isotonic saline infused via a nasogastric tube, or the oral ingestion of a mannitol solution (100 g in 1 litre of water) (this latter regimen should not be used for colonoscopy if diathermy polypectomy is to be used as there is then an increased risk of an explosion).

Any regimen should be modified if there is any evidence of obstruction or active inflammatory bowel disease.

Orally administered non-absorbable antibiotics have now been superseded by intravenous prophylactic antibiotics.

Anaesthesia (general or local)

The decision as to which form of anaesthesia is most appropriate may depend on:

- The procedure
- The patient (see ASA grading below)
- The preference of the anaesthetist and/or surgeon.

The American Society of Anaesthetists grading (ASA) relates patient fitness to outcome after anaesthesia but takes no account of age:

I Normal healthy individual
II Mild systemic disease
III Severe, but not incapacitating, systemic disease
IV Incapacitating systemic disease constantly threatening life
V Moribund patient not expected to survive 24 hours irrespective of intervention
E Suffix for emergency surgery.

General anaesthesia
- With or without full muscle relaxation
- With or without endotracheal intubation
- With or without positive pressure ventilation.

Local anaesthesia
- E.g. 1% or 2% lignocaine
- With or without adrenalin (adrenalin should not be used with lignocaine in the digits or in any area where vasoconstriction may lead to ischaemia.
- Permitted doses are given in Table 13.1.
- Doses may be calculated by knowing that a 1% solution contains 10 mg/ml. Therefore: 20 ml of a 1% solution contains 200 mg; 40 ml of a 0.5% solution contains 200 mg.

Special techniques
- Epidural: A Tuohy needle is used to introduce 6–20 ml of marcaine 0.25–0.5% into the epidural space. This gives a lumboabdominal block, which, although it takes time to establish, can be topped up via a cannula. Opiates, such as 2 mg morphine, are currently used in this manner.
- Spinal: A 22–25 size needle is used to enter the subarachnoid space. After CSF is drawn, 3 ml of 0.5% marcaine or 1.5 ml cinchocaine are introduced. It is a useful technique for quick anaesthesia, but is not suitable for long-term purposes, as a cannula cannot be left in the subarachnoid space for fear of infection. Its onset takes about 10 minutes and lasts for about 1.5 hours.
- Caudal: This route provides ideal analgesia in children for circumcision or herniae. The injection is made via the sacral hiatus, but is not so popular in adults as the hiatus is closed in 10–15%, and large doses are necessary for effective anaesthesia.
- Regional block: This technique is particularly appropriate for day-case herniorrhaphies, e.g. ilio-inguinal block at the anterior superior iliac spine, combined with local infiltration and an injection into the neck of the sac.

Table 13.1

Drug	Plain solution (mg)	With adrenalin (mg)
Lignocaine	200	500
Prilocaine	400	600
Bupivicaine	150	200

- Bier's block: This is especially valuable for setting Colles' fractures. A cuff is placed around the upper arm, and a butterfly needle placed in both arms, one for access to the circulation (on the good hand) and the other to instill the anaesthesia. After elevation, the cuff is inflated and 20–30ml of 0.5% prilocaine injected. 0.2% marcaine has been used but has been known to cause cardiac arrests. The cuff should not be deflated in less than 20 minutes, after which the agent is fixed to the tissues. After the cuff is deflated, a careful watch is made for any signs of toxicity.

Monitoring
- Pulse oximeter (although there is no real alternative to careful clinical observation)
- ECG
- Blood pressure
  — Von Recklinghausen's oscillotenometer
  — automatic blood pressure devices, e.g. dinamap
- Central venous pressure
- Arterial pressure line
- Swan–Ganz balloon catheter to measure pulmonary artery wedge pressure.

Special requirements of anaesthesia
- No muscle relaxants if using the nerve stimulator at parotidectomy
- For bowel anastomoses avoid using neostigmine or atropine, or use them sparingly and carefully
- Thoracic surgery usually requires a double lumen endotracheal tube such as the Carlen or Robert Shaw tube. High-frequency jet ventilation is a useful advance, especially when dealing with a bronchopleural fistula, as the lungs do not go in and out, owing to a small tidal volume, with a high ventilatory rate.
- A bloodless field is vital for neurosurgical procedures, like clipping a berry eneurysm, plastic surgery and some ENT surgery. It is also useful during prostatectomy, parotidectomy and hip replacements. It requires a good premed and deep anaesthesia, and, if the pressure is still too high, beta-blockers will control cardiac rate and hydralazine will lead to vasodilatation. The more powerful sodium nitroprusside must be used carefully as it produces cyanide, and therefore must only be used up to a maximum dose of 1.5 mg/kg body weight.

Position on the table

- Supine: flat on the table and face up, e.g. routine abdominal surgery
- Prone: flat on the table and face down, e.g. excision of a pilonidal sinus
- Lithotomy: hips fully flexed and feet supported on lithotomy poles, e.g. transurethral surgery
- Lloyd Davies: hips semi-flexed and abducted with calves supported on Lloyd Davies stirrups and a sand bag under the sacrum, e.g. abdominoperineal resection of the rectum
- Lateral: full lateral with table broken, e.g. nephrectomy
- Semilateral, e.g. thoracoabdominal approach.

Position of the table

- Head up (reversed Trendelenberg), e.g. to empty veins for head and neck surgery such as thyroidectomy or parotidectomy
- Head down (Trendelenberg), e.g. anterior resection and other pelvic surgery
- Table tilted laterally, e.g. to improve access in certain thoracic procedures.

Skin preparation

Possible solutions for skin preparation

- Chlorhexidine 0.5% in 70% alcohol with or without a dye
- Betadine: povidone-iodine 10% in alcohol
- Aqueous solutions for use in open wounds, face, genitalia, etc.:
  — chlorhexidine 0.15 g/l in cetrimide 1.5 g/l
  — chlorhexidine 0.2 g/l in water.

Describe the drapes and their attachment — towel clips or sutures (avoid towel clips being in the field of view of intraoperative radiology, e.g. operative cholangiography).

Other forms of wound protection:

- Op-site
- Vidrape wound protectors
- Steridrape.

Incisions (Fig. 13.1)

Open surgery

All incisions should be described in relation to specific surface markings. You may be required actually to draw the incision on a model.

Point out any specific hazard or requirements of the incision, e.g.:

- Avoid the marginal/mandibular branch of the facial nerve when making the incision for excision of the submandibular gland
- Include a cephalad extension of the lower abdominal incision for an anterior resection for mobilization of the splenic flexure.

Describe the various layers that are encountered, e.g.:

- Skin
- Subcutaneous fat
- Deep fascia
- Aponeurosis
- Muscle
- Peritoneum, etc.

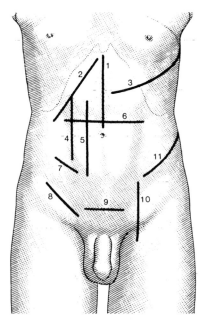

1	Midline
2	Kocher's
3	Thoracoabdominal
4	Rectus split
5	Paramedian
6	Transverse
7	McBurney's gridiron
8	Inguinal
9	Pfannenstiel
10	McEvedy
11	Rutherford Morison

Fig. 13.1 Abdominal incisions.

Laparoscopic surgery

For each laparoscopic procedure describe:

- Patient position and theatre set-up
- Instrument check, e.g. insufflator, camera
- Insertion of first port and induction of pneumoperitoneum
  — open insertion (Hassan) — now most surgeons' preferred
  method
  — Verres needle use
- Secondary port insertions — sizes and sites
- Potential hazards of insertion
- Special instrument or equipment requirements, e.g. specimen
  retrieval bag, staplers, retractors, intraoperative ultrasound.

Initial assessment

Describe any factors that may influence the procedure in hand, e.g.:

- Liver metastases
- Peritoneal seedlings
- Anatomical abnormalities, especially in the biliary tree
- Severe intraperitoneal adhesions
- Synchronous dual pathology.

All intra-abdominal procedures, especially those for trauma, must
include a full laparotomy. It is vital to have a formal sequence for
this procedure in order to avoid omitting any organ from adequate
scrutiny.

Formal laparotomy

A suitable methodical sequence may be as follows:

- Stomach
  — both anterior and posterior aspects
  — open lesser sac
- Pancreas: body and tail can be assessed once lesser sac is open
- Hiatus and diaphragm
  — assess size of hiatus
  — exclude hernia or rupture
- Duodenum
  — Kocherize duodenum — this allows assessment of pancreatic
  head
  — fourth part of duodenum is assessed by reflecting up the
  transverse colon and dividing the ligament of Treitz
- Liver: assess for consistency and presence of masses

- Gall bladder
  — look for stones
  — assess calibre of common bile duct
  — examination with finger in the foramen of Winslow helps assess lower common bile duct and head of pancreas
- Spleen: assess size as well as consistency
- Small bowel
  — look for Meckel's diverticulum
  — mesenteric cysts
  — nodes, tumours or inflammatory lesions
  — vascular abnormalities
- Appendix and caecum: look for faecoliths or tumours
- Colon and rectum
  — look for polyps
  — tumours
  — inflammatory bowel disease
  — diverticular disease
- Pelvic organs
  — uterus
  — tubes
  — ovaries
- Retroperitoneal structures
  — kidneys: size, shape, position
  — ureters: any hold up or dilatation
  — bladder: tumour, stones, diverticulum
  — aorta: aneurysmal dilatation
  — inferior vena cava.

The actual procedure

For each procedure, whether open or laparoscopic, describe:

Mobilization
Give details of the actual anatomical manoeuvres and what instruments are used, i.e.:

- Which retractors, e.g.:
  — Joll's for thyroidectomy
  — Finochieto or Price Thomas for a thoractomy
  — Balfour for a laparotomy
- Any special packing procedure for open procedures, e.g. packing off the hepatic flexure of the colon during cholecystectomy
- What structures are divided or mobilized, e.g.:
  — the peritoneal reflection in a hemicolectomy
  — the strap muscles are separated in a thyroidectomy

Any resection

Give details of margins of resection and define extent of resection
— i.e. for bowel, what clamps are used, e.g.:
  — Lane's twin gastric clamps
  — Hays Lows clamp for anterior resection
  — Zachary Cope's clamp for an end colostomy
- Define extent of resection, e.g.:
  — subtotal thyroidectomy for thyrotoxicosis
  — superficial parotidectomy for pleomorphic ademona
  — limits for a hemicolectomy
- Describe any pedicle ligation, e.g.:
  — renal pedicle: artery before vein to prevent engorgement
  — high inferior mesenteric tie for anterior resection
  — ligation of superior and inferior thyroid arteries during
    thyroidectomy

Intraoperative procedures

— operative cholangiogram during cholecystectomy
— on-table arteriogram after vascular reconstruction
— on-table radiology to assess completeness of nephrolithotomy
— use of nerve stimulator during superficial parotidectomy

Reconstruction

Describe methods of anastomosis and materials used:

- Anterior resection, e.g. end-to-end anastomosis using a single
  layer of interrupted vicryl sutures, prolene, staples, etc.
- Gastric anastomosis, e.g. using two layers of haemostatic
  continuous absorbable sutures such as polyglycolic acid
- Continuous single layer of prolene for vascular anastomoses
- Closing mesentery during bowel resection
- Closing lateral space after colostomy formation.

Potential hazards and their prevention

Point out any particular hazards to the procedure described and also
describe what measures you would take to avoid them, e.g.:

- Laparoscopic procedures present the potential hazards of
  damaging bowel or vessels during port insertion. Specific
  hazards regarding diathermy are considered on page 135.
- At right hemicolectomy you need to avoid damage to the
  ureter and duodenum while the right colic vein can easily
  be torn.

- At superficial parotidectomy you need to avoid damage to the facial nerve. Careful use of the nerve stimulator, scrupulous haemostasis, and patient, painstaking technique, often with operating loops, should help avoid such damage.
- The recurrent laryngeal nerve is easily damaged during thyroidectomy when the inferior thyroid artery region is being dissected. Some surgeons seek to avoid damage by not actively looking for the nerve. However, the author believes the nerve should always be displayed whenever possible.
- The tail of the pancreas can be damaged when ligating the splenic vessels, especially during emergency splenectomy.

Closure of the wound

Describe the wound or port site closure:

- Layers to be closed, e.g.:
  — peritoneum
  — muscle layer: linea alba
  — subcutaneous tissue
  — skin
- Suture materials used, e.g.:
  — nylon
  — prolene
  — catgut
  — dexon
  — vicryl, etc.
- Form of suture, e.g.:
  — interrupted
  — vertical mattress suture
  — deep tension suture
  — subcuticular suture
  — steristrips, etc.

It must be realized that the method of closing wounds becomes an individual matter of preference, as far as both technique and suture material are concerned. However, mass closure of a laparotomy is now the most widely accepted technique, using non-absorbable monofilament nylon, taking large bites of tissue and using plenty of suture length (suture length at least four times the length of the wound).

For any anastomosis or wound closure, tension is anathema and must be avoided at all costs, especially in procedures like mastectomy or amputation flaps.

Drains

Describe any drains used in the procedure. This is again a matter of individual preference, but in deciding which type of drain to use you need to consider:

- What is it draining?
  — air, e.g. underwater seal chest drain
  — blood
  — pus
  — potential contamination, e.g. cystic duct, bowel anastomosis
  — urine
- How long should it be left in and why?
  — until it stops draining
  — 24 hours
  — 5 days
- How should it be managed postoperatively?
  — suction (redivac, sterivac)
  — low-pressure suction, e.g. Roberts pump
  — underwater seal (chest drain)
  — free drainage into dressing
  — free drainage into closed system
  — shortened daily
- How should it be removed?
  — by shortening daily until it falls out
  — removed completely after a certain period of time
  — removed after a sinogram.

Postoperative management

You may be required to give practical advice as to how the patient is managed postoperatively.

General factors
- Postoperative pain relief
- Fluid replacement
- Electrolyte requirements
- Blood replacement
- Physiotherapy to the chest
- General monitoring, i.e.:
  — pulse
  — temperature
  — blood pressure
  — urinary output

— nasogastric aspirate
— other drainage, etc.

Specific factors

These will depend on the procedure:

- Thyroidectomy
  - watch for evidence of:
    - haemorrhage
    - tracheal compression
  - monitor serum calcium
  - check cords
- Vascular surgery
  - watch drainage
  - check limbs for pulses, temperature, capillary return
- Prostatectomy
  - monitor urinary output
  - management of:
    - urinary catheter
    - intracystic irrigation
- Gastrointestinal surgery: nasogastric tube
  - free drainage?
  - 4-hourly aspiration?
  - spigatted?
  - oral fluid restriction

Potential postoperative complications

Causes of operative failure

Pre-operative factors
- Faulty selection of cases
- Poor pre-operative preparation of patient
- Pre-existing intercurrent disease, e.g. myocardial ischaemia, poor respiratory reserve.

Operative factors
- Poor technique, e.g. anastomoses
- Poor haemostasis
- Damage to adjacent organs
- Poor judgement
- Inadequate materials, e.g. sutures
- Poor tissues, e.g. post-irradiation, ischaemia
- Contamination and infection.

Postoperative factors
- Pulmonary atelectasis (collapse)
- Infection: intraperitoneal, wound, etc.
- Chronic cough
- Inadequate management of fluid balance and electrolytes.

Complications of surgery

Anaesthetic
- Inadequate airway
- Inadequate ventilation
- Inadequate fluid replacement
- Inadequate reversal of anaesthetic agents
- Problems resulting from monitoring techniques, e.g. pneumothorax from subclavian venous line, distal ischaemia from arterial line.

Surgical
- Haemorrhage
  — primary (ligature slip, etc.)
  — secondary (infection)
  — reactionary (postoperative rise in blood pressure)
- Poor technique, etc. (see above).

Postoperative

Site
- General, e.g.:
  — pulmonary collapse
  — deep vein thrombosis
  — pulmonary embolism
  — urinary retention
  — metabolic sequelae
- Local, e.g.:
  — haemorrhage
  — infection: wound, etc.
  — specific to that procedure, e.g. post-thyroidectomy:
    — tracheal compression from bleed
    — hypocalcaemia
    — cord malfunction.

Timing
- Immediate (within 24 hours of surgery)
- Early (within 2–3 weeks of surgery)
- Late (remote from surgery).

For full example of postoperative complications, see page 110.

Summary

1. Pre-operative preparation
2. Anaesthesia
3. Position on table
4. Skin preparation
5. Incision
6. Initial assessment
7. Actual procedure
8. Potential hazards and how to avoid them
9. Closure of the wound
10. Drains
11. Postoperative management
12. Potential postoperative complications.

Instruments

It is vital to know the names of specific instruments used in operative procedures, e.g.:

- Retractors
- Clamps
- Forceps
- Purpose-designed instruments.

The examiner may have a selection of instruments in common use available for the candidate to comment on, and he may wish to know:

- What they are called
- What they are used for
- How they are used.

There are a vast number of surgical instruments and those used in any procedure will vary from hospital to hospital according to availability. However, for any particular operation, describe the instruments *you* would use for each specific manoeuvre.

Do not forget to describe the types of suture or ligature used for each manoeuvre.

Suture materials and needles

Suture material is:

1. Absorbable
   - Monofilament
     — plain catgut: tensile strength 21 days

— chromic catgut (chroming slows the rate of absorption and reduces tissue reaction) tensile strength 28 days
— polydiaxanone: tensile strength 56 days
- multifilament: polyglycolic acid (dexon, vicryl): tensile strength 30 days, absorption usually complete by 90 days
2. Non-absorbable
- Monofilament
— polyamide-nylon: degrades at a rate of 15–20% per year
— polyethylene
— polypropylene-prolene: remains indefinitely
— stainless steel
— tantulum
— silver
- Multifilament
— silk: usually cannot be found after 2 years
— linen
— braided polyester (mersilene, dacron, terylene)
— braided polyamide.

Table 13.2 – Suture sizes

Metric number (diameter of suture in 0.1 mm)	Catgut	Non-absorbable
0.1	–	–
0.2	–	10/0
0.3	–	9/0
0.4	–	8/0
0.5	8/0	7/0
0.7	7/0	6/0
1	6/0	5/0
1.5	5/0	4/0
2	4/0	3/0
3	3/0	2/0
3.5	2/0	0
4	0	1
5	1	2
6	2	3 + 4
7	3	5
8	4	6

Needles

Needles are either eyeless (atraumatic) or with eyes for loading separately.

- Round-bodied needles
  — separate tissues rather than cut them
  — after passage of the needle the tissue closes tightly round the suture material, assisting a leak-proof suture line – e.g. intestinal or vascular surgery
  — blunt needles are a variant designed to eliminate needle stick injury and accidental glove puncture
- Round-bodied cutting needles
  — trocar point needles with strong cutting head which increases power of penetration, even into dense tissue
  — tapercut needles combine the initial penetration of a cutting needle with the minimal trauma of a round-bodied needle
- Cutting needles
  — conventional needles have a triangular cross-section
  — extra-cutting needles are tough strong needles with cutting edges extending from the point along half the length of the needle
  — super-cutting needles for skin closure have a modified point profile to obtain maximum incisive penetration
  — reverse cutting needles are triangular in cross-section, with the apex cutting edge on the outside of the needle's curvature
- Colts needle
  — a large hand-held needle that can be threaded separately.

Stapling devices

It is advisable not to suggest to the examiner that such devices are the preferred method of anastomosis, as he is likely to feel that a surgical trainee should be more concerned at improving his suturing technique. However, these instruments are in wide use and it is important to be able to recognize them and to be familiar with their potential value as well as their limitations.

The stapling devices in common use include those for:

- End-to-end anastomoses
- Transverse anastomoses
- Intraluminal anstomoses
- Ligation and division of vessels

- Closure of fascia and skin
- Endoscopic/laparoscopic devices.

Diathermy

Introduction

Short-wave diathermy has proved one of the most versatile and valuable aids to surgical technique. Its most common use is in securing haemostasis by means of coagulation, but by variation of the strength or wave form of the current it can produce a cutting effect, which is particularly employed in transurethral resection in urological surgery or polypectomy via an endoscope in the gastro-intestinal tract.

The principle of diathermy

The patient acts as part of an electrical circuit, and the heat produced depends on:

1. The intensity of the current
2. The wave form of the current
3. The electrical property of the tissues through which the current passes
4. The relative sizes of the two electrodes.

The current

An alternating current is produced by a suitable generator and passed via the active electrode to the patient, through the tissues, and then via a large surface plate (the indifferent electrode) back to the earthed pole of the generator. The amount of heat produced at the active electrode is proportional to the intensity of the current.

The electrode

The other factor affecting heat production is the relative sizes of the electrodes. When a current of high frequency is passed through the body, the tissues between are subjected to heat. If the electrodes are of equal size the heating effect underneath each electrode will also be equal. However, if one electrode is a fine point and the other a large plate (Fig. 13.2), then the heat will be concentrated at the fine point of the active electrode and result in coagulation.

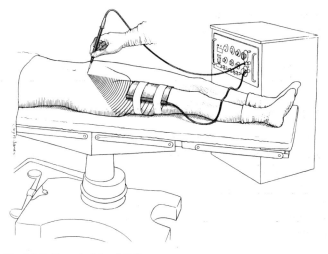

Fig. 13.2 The principle of diathermy.

The tissues

Fat is a poor conductor, but the general passage of the current through the body is by means of the electrolyte solution in the extra-cellular tissues, bloodstream and muscle, which is a good conductor. Skin is a variable conductor, but is a much better one when moistened.

The effects of diathermy

1. Coagulation: sealing off blood vessels.
2. Fulguration: destructive coagulation of tissue with charring, e.g. growth of bladder/rectum.
3. Cutting: used to divide tissues during 'bloodless surgery'.

In the past, 'spark-gap' diathermy produced interrupted bursts of current suitable for coagulation, while 'valve' diathermy produced a purer current of sine wave form causing arcing and division of the tissues (cutting). Blending diathermies could allow both 'spark-gap' coagulation and 'valve' cutting, and the two forms could be simultaneously blended. Today, solid state transistorized diathermy machines are much more reliable and less bulky, and can produce a blended current by being set halfway between the pure sinewave for cutting and the interrupted short bursts for coagulation.

Monopolar and bipolar diathermy (Fig. 13.3A, B)

In *monopolar diathermy*, the most commonly used form, the surgeon uses an active electrode with a very small surface area of contact that concentrates a powerful current at the tip, thus producing heat at the operative point of contact. This is because the power density is very high at this site. The large surface area electrode, the patient plate, completes the circuit and spreads the current over a wide area, thus diminishing the power intensity to such a low level that virtually no heat is produced at this site (Fig. 13.3A). In *bipolar diathermy* the two active electrodes are usually represented by the two limbs of a pair of diathermy forceps. Both forceps ends are active and thus current flows between them, and the heating occurs in the tissue held between the limbs of the forceps (Fig. 13.3B). This form of diathermy is used when it is essential for the surrounding tissue to be free from the risk of either being burned or having the current passing through (e.g. parotid surgery to preserve the facial nerve or circumcision to prevent the complication of channelling — see below).

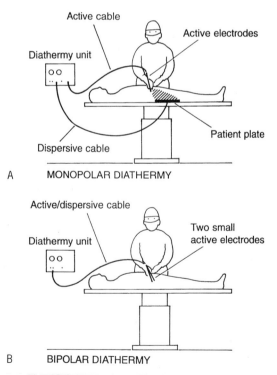

A   MONOPOLAR DIATHERMY

B   BIPOLAR DIATHERMY

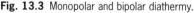

Fig. 13.3 Monopolar and bipolar diathermy.

Complications

Explosion
Sparks can ignite any volatile inflammable gas in the theatre, e.g. ether.

Spirit burns
Inflammable spirit used for preparation of the skin may ignite if the diathermy is used before the spirit has evaporated — e.g. pooling in the umbilicus.

Diathermy burns

- Faulty application of the indifferent electrode may cause an inadequate contact area and therefore cause a local burn
- If the patient touches any other metal object, then he or she is likely to be earthed, e.g.:
  — feet touching the Mayo table
  — arms touching bar of anaesthetic screen
  — hand touching exposed arm rest
  — leg touching naked metal stirrup
- Faulty insulation of diathermy leads, e.g.:
  — towel clips pinching cable
  — cracked insulation
- Inadvertent activity, e.g.:
  — accidental activation of foot pedal
  — accidental contact of active electrode with retractors, instruments, towel clips, etc.

Channelling
Heat is produced where the current intensity is greatest. This is normally at the fine tip of the active electrode, but if current passes up a narrow channel or pedicle, the heat produced may be enough to coagulate these tissues. This can prove disastrous; for example:

- Coagulation of the penis in a child during circumcision
- Coagulation of the spermatic cord when the electrode is applied to the testis.

In such situations diathermy should not be used or, if it is needed, bipolar diathermy should be employed.

Laparoscopic surgery
Inadvertent diathermy burns are a particular hazard of laparoscopic surgery. Such burns might occur in the following ways:

- Diatherming the wrong structure because of lack of clarity of vision or misidentification of structures

- Inadvertent activation of the diathermy pedal while diathermy tip is out of site
- Faulty insulation of laparoscopic equipment
- Intraperitoneal instrument-to-instrument contact while activating diathermy (direct coupling)
- Retained heat in diathermy tip touching structures, e.g. bowel
- Capacitance coupling. This is an unusual phenomenon in which a capacitor is created by having an insulator sandwiched between two electrodes. This can be created by the core of a diathermy 'hook' acting as one electrode and a metal laparoscopic port acting as another electrode with a layer of insulation between them (Fig. 13.4). By means of electromagnetic induction, a diathermy current flowing through an active 'hook' can induce a current in a metal port which can potentially damage intraperitoneal structures. Fortunately such disasters are uncommon, and indeed can be prevented by using plastic ports.

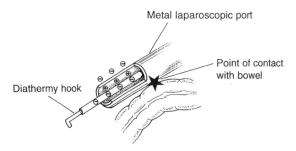

Fig. 13.4 Capacitance coupling.

Prophylactic antibiotics

Prophylactic use of antibiotics in potentially contaminated wounds is now accepted surgical practice. However, the use of such agents depends on both the clinical and bacteriological potential for such contamination.

Clinical potential for infection

- Clean: no breach of a mucosal surface, no local soiling, e.g. thyroidectomy
- Clean-contaminated: mucosal surface breached but procedure is clean, e.g. cholecystectomy

- Contaminated: a viscus containing large quantities of bacteria is entered, e.g. elective colorectal surgery
- Dirty: the wound is exposed to pus or infected visceral contents, e.g. colonic perforation.

Bacteriological potential for infection

This is defined by visceral and parietal swabs taken during the operation. The potential for infection in any wound is defined by the results of the swabs allowing for the classification presented.

- Clean: both visceral and parietal swabs sterile
- Potentially contaminated: visceral swab contaminated, parietal swab sterile
- Lightly contaminated: a single species grown from parietal swab
- Heavily contaminated: two or more species grown from parietal swab

It is vital to stress that the use of prophylactic antibiotics is in no way a substitute for scrupulous surgical and aseptic technique, but merely an adjunct. Other factors that affect the risk of sepsis include procedures of longer than 2 hours' duration, the insertion of protheses and any existing intercurrent disease process (e.g. rheumatic valve disease) or relevant medication (e.g. steroids). The use of such agents raises certain practical clinical questions.

When should they be given?
Prophylactic antibiotics are ineffective unless circulating within 2 or 3 hours of contamination. Therefore, the first dose should be given immediately before surgery — most conveniently at induction of anaesthesia.

Which antibiotics?
This depends on the potential bacterial contamination. With new antibiotics being frequently presented on the market it is impossible to be dogmatic, but as a general rule a broad-spectrum antibiotic like the cephalosporins is commonly used for upper abdominal surgery, combined with an anti-anaerobic agent like metronidazole for colorectal surgery. Some of the newer generation of antibiotics have both anti-aerobic and anti-anaerobic activity, and may be suitable for single-agent prophylaxis in this context.

For how long should it be given?
Initial evidence suggested that three doses were adequate for prophylaxis, although more recent evidence suggests that one dose only

may be effective and sufficient. However, if a procedure is prolonged, with a duration of over 2 hours, then a further dose may be indicated. There is certainly no indication that more than three doses will provide any further protection as far as prophylaxis is concerned, but when one is treating an established infection — e.g. perforated diverticular disease — a longer course is usually necessary; but this then falls into the therapeutic category of 'treatment' rather than prophylaxis.

By which route?
Both intravenous or intra-incisional administration have proved effective in different series. Intravenous administration at the time of anaesthetic induction is most commonly used in everyday current practice. Rectal metronidazole has proved adequate prophylaxis for appendicectomy.

What are the potential problems?
- It may encourage the emergence of resistant strains, but this can be limited by limiting the course of antibiotics to a one- or three-dose regimen.
- Even one dose may cause later anaphylaxis.

Thromboembolic prophylaxis

Any patient undergoing surgical procedures is at risk of developing thromboembolic complications owing to the hypercoagulable state that is a component of the body's metabolic response to stress. This is exacerbated by underlying malignancy, sepsis, trauma, dehydration and emergency surgery. A past history of a thromboembolic episode, increasing age, obesity and a prolonged operative procedure also increase the risk.

Prophylactic methods in current use
- Graded compression stockings (TED stockings). A good fit is required, and there should be no history of peripheral vascular disease, with foot pulses present.
- Pneumatic compression boots during surgery
- Subcutaneous heparin (5000 units subcutaneously twice daily). This acts by inactivation of thrombin and factor Xa by enhancement of antithrombin III activity. Newer low-molecular-weight heparins inactivate factor Xa only, and need to be administered only once a day (e.g. enoxaprin 20–40 mg sc od).

Possible protocol for use

Risk	Risk factors	Prophylaxis
High	Past history of deep vein thrombosis, pulmonary embolism or cerebrovascular accident (beware of CVA bleed) Major pelvic or abdominal surgery Surgery for malignancy	Compression boots TED stockings Heparin sc
Moderate	Patient > 40 years Surgery > 30 minutes On oral contraceptive Relevant intercurrent disease	Heparin sc TED stockings
Low	Patient < 40 years Surgery < 30 minutes No additional risk factors	Early mobilization

Additional risk factors include:

- Obesity
- Varicose veins
- Pregnancy
- Immobility
- Hypercoagulable states
- Recent surgery
- Sepsis
- Dehydration
- Trauma or emergency surgery.

Endoscopy

Diagnostic

- Oesophagoscopy
- Gastroscopy
- Duodenoscopy
- Endoscopic-retrograde-cholangio-pancreatography (ERCP)
- Choledochoscopy
- Colonoscopy
- Cystoscopy
- Nephroscopy
- Laparoscopy
- Arthroscopy
- Bronchoscopy.

Biopsy and cytology facilities are available with all the above techniques.

Therapeutic

- Dilatation of strictures
- Injection of oesophageal varices
- Oesophageal intubation
- Control of haemorrhage
  — diathermy
  — resin glues
  — laser
- Removal of foreign bodies
- Endoscopic papillotomy
- Endoscopic polypectomy
- Removal of retained common bile duct stones
- Arthroscopic meniscectomy
- Laparoscopic surgery: minimal access surgery, e.g. cholecystectomy, fundoplication, laparoscopically assisted colectomy, etc.

Complications

- Perforation
- Haemorrhage following:
  — papillotomy
  — polypectomy
  — laparoscopic procedures
- Cross-infection
- Explosion (when using diathermy in colon with mannitol used as bowel preparation)
- Specific
  — acute pancreatitis after ERCP
  — complications of laparoscopic surgery
    — direct damage at port insertion
      — blood vessels
      — bowel
      — other intraperitoneal structures, e.g. liver
    — pneumoperitoneum
      — gas embolism
      — splinting diaphragm
      — surgical emphysema
    — diathermy damage (see p. 135)
    — direct damage during dissection

— haemorrhage
— structural damage, e.g. common bile duct
— inadvertent damage by any mechanism.

Finally...

Thomas' Golden Rules for 'Perfect' Surgery

- The *right* operation on the *right* side of the *right* patient at the *right* time
- Absolute asepsis
- Adequate exposure (includes the siting of incisions and laparoscopic ports)
- Immaculate operative technique
- Scrupulous haemostasis.

If these rules are carefully followed, then if anything goes wrong it is the fault of the pathology, the patient or maybe even the anaesthetist!

Applied physiology and critical care

14

During this viva you will be asked about clinically relevant physiological matters, especially those relating to the management of surgical patients or patients in an intensive care unit. The first 10 minutes with a physiologist will cover physiology with prompts such as clinical charts, results, X-rays, ECGs, etc. The second 10 minutes with a surgeon will cover critical care and emergencies.

Many of the topics are to a degree predictable, and although the following subjects are in no way a complete review of what could be asked, they certainly represent topics that are commonly asked.

Intensive care units (including high dependency)

ITU

An area patients are admitted to when they require:

- Treatment for actual or impending organ failure
- Mechanical ventilation
- Specific specialty requirements
  — neurosurgical
  — renal
  — paediatric.

HDU

An area patients are admitted to when they require:

- Intensive observation
- Intensive nursing
- Invasive monitoring.

Consider:

- Their structure and financing
  - design, e.g.:
    - room for bulky equipment
    - isolation facilities
    - ? 25% of beds as cubicles
    - adequate oxygen, electricity, etc.
  - location, e.g.:
    - near to source of patients (A & E, theatres)
    - support services, e.g. radiology
    - grouped together i.e. ITU, HDU, CCU
  - staff
    - nursing
    - medical
    - training programmes
- Their day-to-day management: scoring systems, e.g.:
  - APACHE (acute physiology and chronic health evaluation)
  - SAPS (simplified acute physiology score)
  - TISS (therapeutic intervention scoring system)
- Complications, e.g.:
  - psychological impact on:
    - patients
    - relatives
    - staff
  - cross-infection
- Cost-effectiveness, i.e.:
  - daily costs of ITU are approximately three times the cost of a regular hospital stay
  - outcome data.

Also consider the following aspects of management:

- Ventilation
- Monitoring
- Fluid balance and dialysis
- Nutrition
- Blood transfusion.

Ventilation

Adequate tissue oxygenation depends upon:

- Airway
- Breathing
- Circulation.

Respiratory failure

There are two patterns:

Type I (hypoxaemic)
- PaO_2 reduced with normal or reduced $PaCO_2$
- Ventilation/perfusion mismatch, e.g.:
  — pulmonary embolism
  — cyanotic heart disease
  — adult respiratory distress syndrome (ARDS)

Type II (ventilatory)
- PaO_2 reduced and $PaCO_2$ elevated
- Impaired gas exchange due to defect in mechanics of breathing
  — impaired central control, e.g.:
    — head injuries
    — drugs
  — inadequate chest movement, e.g.
    — paralysis: cervical spine injuries
    — trauma: disruption of chest wall integrity
    — pain
    — diaphragmatic splinting: intestinal obstruction
    — deformity: cicatrizing burns
  — reduced lung volume, e.g.:
    — pneumothorax
    — atelectasis
    — consolidation
    — contusion.

Oxygen delivery

- Humidified
- Low-flow oxygen
  — nasal cannulae or simple masks
  — oxygen flow of 4 l/min
  — can provide inspired oxygen concentration (F_iO_2) of 30–40%
  — used for patients relying on hypoxic drive to breathe
- High-flow oxygen
  — needs special masks
  — used for patients with a pulmonary shunt (V/P mismatch)
  — can achieve F_iO_2 of up to 60%
- Continuous positive airway pressure (CPAP)
  — mask with tight seal

— facilitates opening of collapsed alveoli
— helps disperse pulmonary oedema
- Positive end expiratory pressure (PEEP)
  — used during mechanical ventilation
  — similar effect to CPAP
  — may reduce cardiac output by impaired venous return
- Mechanical ventilation
  — indications
    — respiratory failure not correctable by conservative means
    — raised intracranial pressure
    — patients at risk of postoperative fatigue
    — inability to protect airway
    — the need for multiple surgical procedures: 'second looks'
  — tracheostomy
    — required after endotracheal intubation for 10 days
    — allows good bronchial toilet
    — minitracheostomy satisfactory for short-term use
    — permanent after radical larynx/pharynx surgery
    — often required after head and neck trauma
    — reduces dead space.

Lung function tests

Peak expiratory flow rate (PEFR)

- Peak flow gauge or Wright's peak flow meter
- Measures peak expiratory flow in litres/minute in first 1/100 second
- Assesses severity of airflow obstruction.

Forced expiratory volume in 1 second (FEV$_1$)

- Measured by dry wedge spirometry
- Correlates well with PEFR
- $FEV_1/PEFR = > 10$ (Empey index) decreased in large airways obstruction.

Forced vital capacity (FVC)

- Measured by spirometry
- Decreased in restrictive pattern of disease
- Useful for reduced lung volume or chest wall problems
- $FEV_1/FVC < 70\%$ indicates airways obstruction.

Blood gases

- Transcutaneous pulse oximetry
  - measures haemoglobin oxygen saturation (SaO_2)
  - painless and quick
  - unreliable with low tissue perfusion
- PaO_2 (partial pressure of oxygen in arterial blood)
  - requires arterial sampling
  - reflects ventilation/perfusion matching
  - measured in kPa
- $PaCO_2$ (partial pressure of carbon dioxide in arterial blood)
  - reflects ventilation
  - transcutaneous CO_2 monitors fast and painless
  - can identify those at risk of underventilation.

Monitoring

Non-invasive

- Pulse rate
- Blood pressure
- ECG
- Temperature
- Respiratory rate
- Urine output
- Fluid balance
- Pulse oximetry

Invasive

- CVP
  - measures pressure in right atrium and great veins
  - normal range is wide (0–10 mmHg, 1–12 cm H_2O)
  - changes in CVP better guide than single readings
  - access via
    - internal jugular vein, preferably right side
    - subclavian vein
    - cephalic or femoral vein
  - complications of central venous cannulation
    - puncture of apical pleura: pneumothorax
    - bleeding and haematoma
    - air embolus

- — catheter infection
- — thrombophlebitis
- — erosion of catheter tip through right atrium (rare)
- Arterial blood pressure
  - — peripheral arterial cannulation
  - — radial artery preferred site
- Pulmonary artery wedge pressure
  - — pulmonary artery flotation catheters, e.g. Swan-Ganz
  - — catheter floated into a branch of the pulmonary artery
  - — 'wedging' measures pulmonary capillary pressure
  - — indicates left atrial pressure
  - — useful estimate of left ventricular end-diastolic pressure
  - — a mortality of up to 2% has been recorded
  - — clearly defined indications for use are necessary, e.g.:
    - — patients with septic or cardiogenic shock
    - — poor left ventricular function after cardiac surgery
    - — pulmonary oedema (indicates nature of cause)
- Cardiac output
- Systemic vascular resistance.

Fluid balance

Water

Percentage of body weight
- Adult man: 60% ⎫ diminishing
- Adult woman: 50% ⎭ with age
- The obese: 45%
- Neonates: 75%

Distribution

	Volume in litres	% of body weight
Total body weight	42	60
Intracellular	28	40
Extracellular	14	20
• Plasma	3	5
• Interstitial	10	14
• Transcellular	1	1

Fluid Balance

Intake (ml)		Output (ml)	
Water from beverages	1200	Urine	1500
Water from food	1000	Insensible loss	900
Water from oxidation	300	Faeces	100
Total	2500	Total	2500

Poor urinary output
- Hypovolaemia
- Acute tubular necrosis
- Urinary retention.

Gastrointestinal tract fluid secretion
- Total turnover: 5–8 l
- Saliva: 300–500 ml
- Gastric juice: 1200–2000 ml
- Bile: 500–1200 ml
- Pancreatic juice: 500–800 ml
- Succus entericus: 2500–3500 ml.

Electrolytes (in mmol/l)

		Intracellular fluid	Serum
Cations	Sodium (Na)	10	140
	Potassium (K)	160	4
	Others	14	2
Anions	Chloride (Cl)	3	102
	Bicarbonate (HCO_3)	10	27
	Phosphate (PO_4)	106	1

Oedema (mechanisms)
- Raised capillary hydrostatic pressure, e.g.:
  — cardiac failure
  — venous obstruction: DVT
- Decreased plasma oncotic pressure, e.g.:
  — nephrotic syndrome
  — liver cirrhosis

- Increased capillary permeability
  - angioneurotic oedema
  - adult respiratory distress syndrome
- Lymphatic obstruction
  - primary lymphoedema
  - malignant infiltration
- Renal sodium retention
  - renal failure
  - glomerulonephritis.

Fluid accumulations

- Exudate
  - > 30 g protein/litre
  - infection
  - lymphatic obstruction
  - malignancy
- Transudate
  - < 30 g protein/litre
  - excess interstitial fluid
  - decreased oncotic presure
  - decreased interstitial fluid resorption.

Dialysis

Indications
- Removal of excess fluid
- Hyperkalaemia
- Acidosis
- Rapidly climbing plasma creatinine

Methods
- Peritoneal dialysis
  - unlikely to be appropriate after emergency surgery
  - continuous ambulatory peritoneal dialysis (CAPD) in chronic cases
  - Tenckhoff permanent peritoneal catheter
  - peritonitis is commonest complication
- Haemodialysis
  - vascular access required, e.g. cannulation, Scribner shunt, A-V fistula
  - countercurrent diffusion across semipermeable membrane
  - can remove large fluid volumes rapidly
  - may not be well tolerated by the critically ill

- Haemofiltration
  - blood is pumped through a filter — filtrate discarded
  - fluid removed continuously at slower rate than haemodialysis
  - causes less cardiovascular disturbance.

Nutrition

Nutritional requirements

- Depends on energy expenditure
- 75% of patients require:
  - 14 g nitrogen
  - 2000 non-nitrogen calories
  - minerals and vitamins
- Hypercatabolic patients require additional support.

Methods

- Enteral
- Parenteral.

Enteral feeding

- Elemental diets
  - L amino acids and sugars
  - relatively expensive
  - unpalatable
  - non-antigenic
  - e.g. used in children with Crohn's disease
- Defined liquid diets
  - peptones, polysaccharides, medium-chain triglycerides
  - vitamins, trace elements, electrolytes
  - osmolality only slightly more than plasma to prevent diarrhoea
- Delivery
  - fine-bore nasoduodenal tubes
  - nasogastric tubes
  - gastrostomy tubes
  - jejunostomy tubes.

Parenteral feeding

Indications
- Absolute: enterocutaneous fistula

- Relative
  - malnutrition
  - multiple trauma
  - oesophagectomy
  - prolonged ileus
  - abdominal sepsis
  - Crohn's disease
  - pancreatitis
  - multisystem failure.

Content
- Standard regimen
  - 14 g nitrogen
  - 250 g glucose
  - 500 ml 20% lipid
  - 100 mmol sodium
  - 70 mmol potassium
  - 10 mmol calcium
  - 140 mmol acetate
  - plus magnesium, zinc, phosphate, vitamins, etc.

Complications
- Of line insertion
  - failure to cannulate
  - pneumothorax
  - hydrothorax
  - arterial puncture
  - brachial plexus injury
  - mediastinal haematoma
  - thoracic duct injury
- Of continuing care
  - septicaemia
  - air embolus
  - thrombosis
  - catheter embolus
  - cardiac tamponade.

Monitoring
- Daily calorie intake
- Weekly weight measurement
- Nitrogen balance assessment (nitrogen excretion g/24 h = urine urea × 24 h urine vol × 0.028 × 6/5)
- Biochemical and haematological indices.

Blood transfusion

Collection and storage

- 450 ml free-flowing venous blood is stored with 63 ml of anticoagulant mixture of citrate, phosphate, dextrose, adenine (CPD-A)
- Kept at ambient temperature for 4 hours to encourage phagocytes and plasma opsonins to eliminate skin bacteria
- Subsequently stored at 4°C for up to 35 days
- Mandatory testing for:
  — antibodies to HIV-1 and HIV-2
  — hepatitis C virus
  — hepatitis B surface antigen
  — syphilis
- Some donations tested for:
  — antibodies to human T cell leukaemia virus, HTLV I and HTLV II
  — hepatitis B core antigen
  — liver enzymes
  — antibodies to Cytomegalovirus (CMV)
- Automated donation grouping for ABO and RhD
- Phenotyping for other blood groups may include:
  — RhC/c or RhE/e
  — Kell
  — Duffy (Fy)
  — Kidd (Jk)
- Compatibility testing:
  — group the patient's blood for ABO and RhD type
  — screen the serum for antibodies
  — save a portion of serum for matching with donor blood as required.

Potential complications

- Febrile reactions
- Allergic reactions
- Circulatory overload
- Haemolytic reactions
  — incompatibility
  — old stored blood
  — haemolysed blood from overheating or freezing
- Infected blood
- Thrombophlebitis

- Air embolus
- Transmission of disease, e.g.
  - hepatitis (HbSAg positive)
  - AIDS
  - malaria
  - syphilis
- Transfusion haemosiderosis
- Massive transfusion
  - cardiac arrhythmias
  - excess citrate
  - hypocalcaemia
  - hyperkalaemia
  - fall in blood pH
  - cold blood.

Sepsis

Definitions

Bacteraemia
Presence of viable bacteria in the blood stream.

Systemic inflammatory response syndrome (SIRS)
Inflammatory response to severe clinical insult

- Temperature > 38°C or < 36°C
- Heart rate > 90/min
- Respiratory rate > 20/min
- White blood cells (WBC) > 12×10^9/litre or < 4×10^9/litre.

Sepsis
SIRS as a result of infection.

Septic shock
Sepsis associated with evidence of tissue hypoperfusion and hypotension

- Metabolic acidosis
- Oliguria
- Mental confusion.

Multiple organ dysfunction syndrome (MODS)
SIRS, sepsis or septic shock associated with impaired organ function

- Respiratory failure

- Renal failure
- Hepatic dysfunction
- Coagulopathy.

Biochemistry

Other discussion topics may centre around the practical interpretation of routine results, e.g. biochemical changes in clinical conditions.

It is wise to have at your fingertips the normal values and ranges of routine biochemical investigations (see Appendix 4), and the changes that can occur in many of the more common or interesting clinical conditions, for example:

Addison's disease

- Serum sodium: low
- Serum potassium: high
- Blood urea nitrogen: high
- Blood glucose: low
- Plasma cortisol fails to rise after intravenous ACTH.

Cirrhosis

- Serum bilirubin: high
- Serum albumin: low
- Serum gamma globulin: high
- Serum sodium: low
- Alanine amino transferase: high
- Aspartate amino transferase: high
- Alkaline phosphatase: raised (not as high as obstructive jaundice)
- Serum cholesterol: high
- Haemoglobin: low
- Prothrombin time: prolonged
- Urinary bilirubin: present.

Conn's syndrome

- Serum aldosterone: high
- Serum potassium: low
- Serum sodium: high
- Blood pH: high
- Urinary aldosterone: high
- Urinary specific gravity: low.

Hyperparathyroidism

- Serum calcium: high
- Serum phosphate: low
- Serum parathormone: inappropriately high
- Alkaline phosphatase: high
- Urinary calcium: high
- Urinary phosphate: high.

Pyloric stenosis

- Dehydrated
- Haematocrit: raised
- Serum sodium: low
- Serum chloride: low
- Serum potassium: low
- Plasma bicarbonate: high
- Plasma urea: high
- Blood pH: high
- Serum ionized calcium: low
- Urine volume: decreased
- Urine pH: initially alkaline, later acid.

Acute renal failure

- Blood urea nitrogen: high
- Serum creatinine: high
- Creatinine clearance: low
- Haemoglobin: low
- Urinary phosphate: high
- Blood pH: low
- Serum potassium: high
- Serum sodium: low.

Many other syndromes can be tackled in the same way, and may well crop up as clinical vignettes, if not in this viva, then in the MCQ question papers, especially the extended matching questions that lend themselves well to this type of data analysis.

Pain control

Postoperative pain

Assessment of pain

- Regular clinical assessment

- Formal assessment (pain charts)
- Functional assessment, e.g.:
  — abdominal wounds
  — chest movements
  — deep breathing.

Drugs
- Opioids, e.g. pethidine, morphine
- Local anaesthetics, e.g. marcaine 0.5%, lignocaine 1–2%
  — infiltration (all layers)
  — nerve blocks, e.g.
    — brachial block
    — intercostal block
    — ulnar nerve block
  — regional, e.g.
    — epidural
    — spinal
    — caudal
- Non-steroidal anti-inflammatory agents, e.g. voltarol.

Routes of administration
- Parenteral
  — intramuscular
  — intravenous (IV)
  — subcutaneous (SC)
  — epidural, e.g. local anaesthetics and/or opioids
- Oral (once the patient is eating and drinking), e.g. voltarol, dihydrocodeine, oromorph, paracetamol
- Rectal, e.g. voltarol.

Methods of administration
- Nurse administered, e.g. intramuscular
- Patient-controlled, e.g.
  — PCA pumps (IV, SC, epidural)
  — oral regimens
- Continuous infusion, e.g.:
  — intravenous
  — subcutaneous
  — epidural.

Potential complications
- Opioids, e.g.:
  — respiratory depression

- — sedation
- — constipation
- — urinary retention
- — itching
- NSAIDs, e.g.:
  - — gastrointestinal irritation
  - — renal failure
  - — antiplatelet
- Local anaesthetics, e.g.:
  - — paraesthesia
  - — anaesthesia (pressure areas)
  - — weakness
- Epidural, e.g.
  - — postural hypotension
  - — urinary retention

Chronic pain control

The relief of chronic intractable pain is vital for the sake of the patient's morale, but can prove extremely difficult in practice. Pain relief clinics have sought not only to highlight the need for such relief, but also to provide a satisfactory practical answer to many of the problems these patients present with. The commonest aetiological factor is back pain, but malignancy, phantom limb pain and causalgia can prove equally as problematic.

The causes of malignancy-induced pain
1. Compression.
2. Pathological fracture.
3. Infiltration of nerves.
4. Visceral obstruction.
5. Vascular obstruction causing ischaemia.
6. Necrosis.
7. Infection and inflammation.
8. Tension by infiltration in restrictive structures.

Therapeutic options in treating intractable pain
- Surgical correction of any mechanical cause if possible; e.g. defunctioning colostomy for irresectable obstructing pelvic malignancy
- Analgesic drugs
  - — orally (often in combination with other drugs)
  - — adequate frequency and dosage are vital

— subcutaneous infusion by pump, e.g. diamorphine
— parenteral: intramuscular or intravenous (most often used at the end-stage of the disease)
— with analgesic drugs it is vital to ensure that pain is relieved by an adequate dose of the prescribed agents, before the effect of the last dose has worn off — i.e. 'by the clock' prescribing rather than 'prn'
- Local nerve blocks, e.g. intercostal nerve blocks with local anaesthetic or neurolytic with alcohol or phenol
- Plexus blocks, e.g. coeliac plexus blocks for inoperable malignancy of pancreas or stomach
- Spinal subarachnoid block, e.g. for pain in abdomen, pelvis and lower limbs (complication with bladder function can occur if sacral nerves are involved and may require catheterization)
- Percutaneous electrical cordotomy (popular in USA but only available in a few centres in Great Britain). Destroys the anterolateral tract at upper end of spinal cord (spinothalamic cordotomy)
- Dorsal column stimulation: self stimulation by the patient by means of a transmitter and subcutaneous implanted receiver button with platignum electrodes. This raises the threshold to pain.

In all forms of pain relief, success will depend on a positive approach, careful assessment and considerable insight into the patient's needs, both physically and psychologically, in order to make the proper selection of patients for each method available.

Radiology

X-rays and scans are a common starting point for discussion. In describing radiographs or scans, however, one must be disciplined, or else vital features on a film may be either missed or inadequately presented.
    When describing a radiograph:

1. What is the X-ray or scan? e.g.:
   - Plain chest X-ray
   - Plain abdominal X-ray
   - Barium meal
   - Barium enema
   - Intravenous urogram
   - Myelogram
   - Ultrasound scan
   - CT scan
   - MRI scan.

2. What is the position and orientation of the X-ray? e.g.:
   - Posterior-anterior view
   - Anterior-posterior view
   - Lateral (left or right)
   - Erect, supine or decubitus.
3. If presented with more than one film, check:
   - Is the name of the patient the same?
   - Is the date the same?
   - Are the films sequential?
4. If presented with a film employing contrast medium:
   - Is a control film available?

Examination of any X-ray needs to be methodical and it is wise to have a sequence for examining and describing the pertinent features displayed.

Chest X-ray

The position of the patient
- Is the patient straight or rotated?
- Look and see if the medial ends of the clavicles are symmetrically related to the vertebral column.

The bony structures
- Is the chest symmetrical?
- Is there a scoliosis?
- Are all the ribs present? (one missing suggests previous surgery)
- Are the ribs unduly crowded or widely spaced in any area?
- Are the ribs
  — notched? (coarctation)
  — eroded? (metastic deposits)
- Are there any fractures?

The trachea
- Is this central or deviated? If deviated, is it pushed or pulled over?
- Is the dark column of air symmetrical or is there any narrowing or compression (Fig. 14.1)?
- Is the carina widened, e.g. secondary metastatic node enlargement?

The heart
- Is the heart outline normal: size, shape, position?
- Is there evidence of a pericardial effusion (large globular heart shadow)?

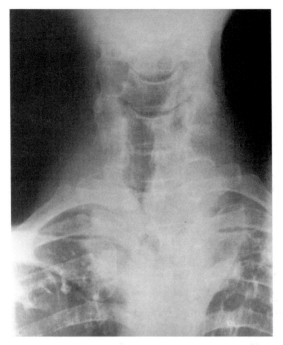

Fig. 14.1 Tracheal compression.

- Is there left ventricular enlargement (boot-shaped heart), e.g. aortic incompetence, aortic stenosis, hypertension?
- Is there left atrial enlargement (convex swelling of the left border of the heart), e.g. mitral stenosis, mitral incompetence? (left atrial enlargement can also be delineated by a right oblique view of a barium swallow)

The mediastinum
- Is the aorta aneurysmal or unfolded?
- Are there any soft tissue shadows, e.g. retrosternal goitre (Fig. 14.2), enlarged thymus, lymph nodes?
- Are there any fluid levels apparent (Fig. 14.3), e.g. hiatus hernia, achalasia, mediastinal abscess?

The diaphragm
- Is the outline clear on both sides?
- Is the outline normal: shape and position?
- Are the cardiophrenic and costophrenic angles clear or is there an effusion (Fig. 14.4)?
- Is there any free air under the diaphragm (Fig. 14.5)?

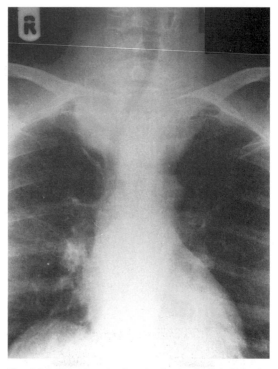

Fig. 14.2 Retrosternal goitre showing tracheal deviation to the right.

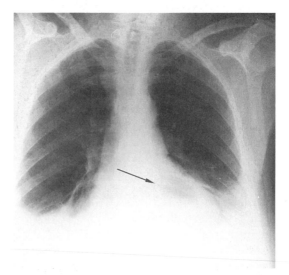

Fig. 14.3 Fluid level behind the heart — a large hiatus hernia.

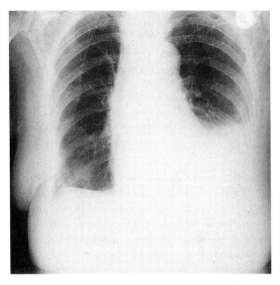

Fig. 14.4 A left-sided pleural effusion.

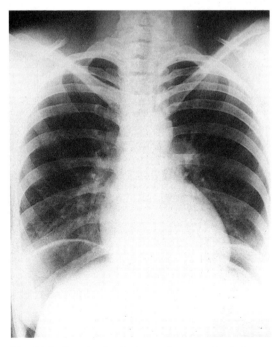

Fig. 14.5 Air under the diaphragm from a perforated duodenal ulcer.

The lungs
- Divide the lung fields into three zones:
  - — upper zone: apex to anterior end of 2nd costal cartilage
  - — mid zone: from anterior end of 2nd costal cartilage to lower border of 4th costal cartilage
  - — lower zone: from lower border of 4th costal cartilage to bases
- Are there any abnormal shadows?
- Are the hilar shadows normal: size and position?
- Are the vascular markings more prominent (pulmonary plethora)?
- Are the vascular markings inconspicuous (pulmonary oligaemia)?
- Are any fissures visible? (the minor interlobar fissure on the right may sometimes be seen in a normal film)
- Are there any Kerley B lines (engorged subpleural lymphatics at lung bases due to raised left atrial pressure)?
- Is there any evidence of a pneumothorax?
- Is one lung field more opaque than the other? (if so, ask for an erect film which may show a large effusion or haemothorax, etc.)

Soft tissue shadows
- Are there any breast shadows, i.e. female patient?
- Are they both present and symmetrical? (if one is missing the patient has had a mastectomy)
- Are there any other extrathoracic soft tissue swellings?

Abdominal X-ray

The position of the patient
- Is the film taken in an erect, supine or in a lateral decubitus position?
- Check the flank stripes and psoas margins for symmetry and normal sharp interfaces.

The penetration of the film
- Is it overpenetrated?
  - — free peritoneal air
  - — large amount of gas in the gut
  - — thin patient.
- Is it underpenetrated?
  - — ascites
  - — obesity
  - — fluid-filled loops of gut
  - — soft tissue masses.

The bony structures

- Are all the ribs present? (an absent 12th rib may indicate previous renal surgery)
- Is the spine normal, or is there evidence of:
  — scoliosis
  — ankylosing spondylitis
  — osteoarthritis with osteophyte formation
  — secondary deposits and/or collapse?
- Is the pelvis normal, or is there evidence of:
  — Paget's disease
  — secondary deposits
  — osteoarthritis of the hips (Fig. 14.6)
  — fractures?

The intestinal gas pattern

- Is it normal?
- Are there any fluid levels (Fig. 14.7)? (in children under 2 years, fluid levels in the small bowel are a normal occurrence)
- More than three fluid levels is regarded as being unphysiological:
  — gastric fundus
  — duodenal cap
  — terminal ileum (rare)
- Are there any distended loops of bowel?

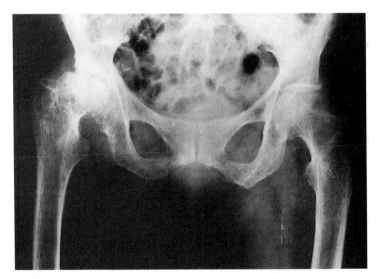

Fig. 14.6 Osteoarthritis of the right hip.

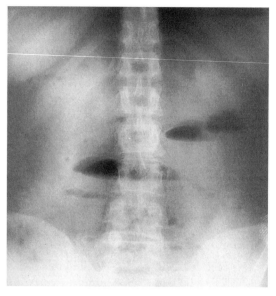

Fig. 14.7 Air/fluid levels in intestinal obstruction.

- Can the loops be identified (Fig. 14.8)? e.g.:
  — jejunum: transverse folds of valvulae conniventes extending across the bowel giving a concertina effect
  — ileum: characterless outline
  — caecum: a rounded blob of gas in right iliac fossa
  — colon: haustral folds that are spaced irregularly and do not traverse the complete width of the bowel
- Is there any uncontained air
  — outside gut
  — in the biliary tree (Fig. 14.9)
  — under the liver or lateral to it
  — under the diaphragm (Fig. 14.5)
  — in abscess cavities
  — in the bladder (pneumaturia, Fig. 14.10)?

Soft tissue shadows
- Are the visible organ masses normal in size?
  — the splenic tip
  — the liver edge
  — the renal outlines
  — the urinary bladder
- Are the psoas shadows present and normal?
- Are there any unexplained soft tissue shadows?

Jejunum   Ileum

Caecum   Colon

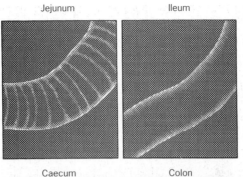
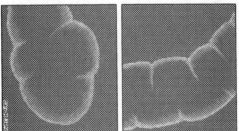

Fig. 14.8 The pattern of distended bowel loops. Typical bowel shadows on plain abdominal radiographs.

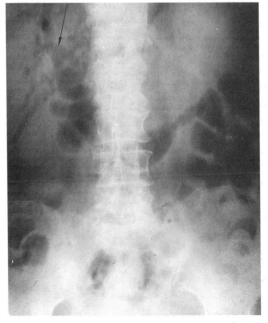

Fig. 14.9 Pneumobilia from a cholecystoduodenal fistula.

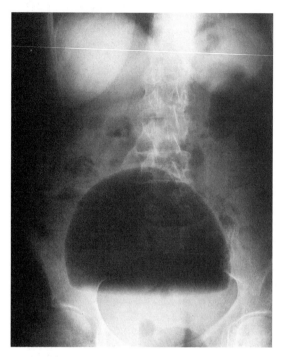

Fig. 14.10 Pneumaturia due to a vesicocolic fistula.

Is there any extraskeletal calcification?

- Rib cartilages
- Vessels
  - — especially aortic, iliac or splenic aneurysms (Fig. 14.11)
  - — phleboliths
- Genitourinary calculi (Fig. 14.12)
- Gallstones (Fig. 14.13) (only 10% of all gallstones are calcified)
- Pancreatic calcification: chronic pancreatitis (Fig. 14.14)
- Mesenteric lymph nodes
- Dermoid cysts.

Limbs and bones

The patient

- Can the patient's maturity be assessed, e.g. epiphyseal fusion (Fig. 14.15)?
- What is the orientation of the X-ray, i.e. which bone and side?
- Are two views available, e.g. anteroposterior, lateral or oblique?
- Are two limbs available for comparison?

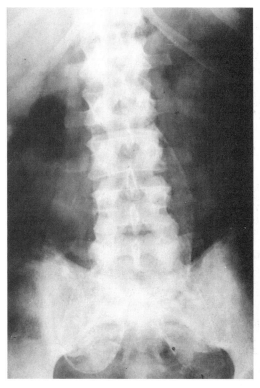

Fig. 14.11 Calcification in the walls of aortic and iliac aneurysms.

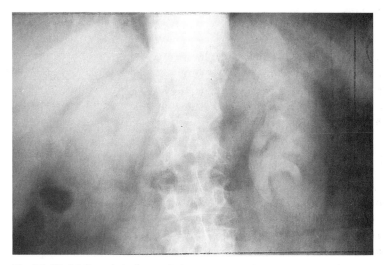

Fig. 14.12 A left renal staghorn calculus.

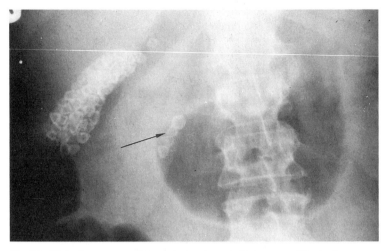

Fig. 14.13 Radio-opaque gallstones (note stones in the common bile duct).

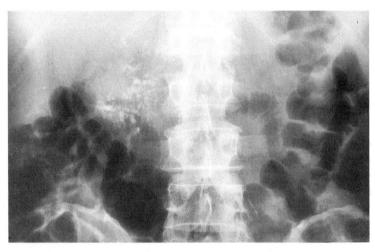

Fig. 14.14 Pancreatic calcification in chronic pancreatitis.

Soft tissues

- Are there any foreign bodies visible?
- Is there any extraosseus calcification? e.g.:
    — haematoma (myositis ossificans)
    — tendon or tendon sheath (peritendonitis calcarea)
    — veins (phleboliths)
- Are there any soft tissue swellings, e.g. tumours, lipomas?

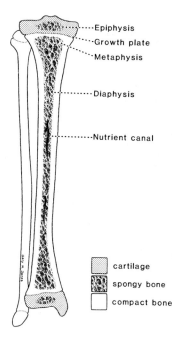

Epiphysis

Growth plate

Metaphysis

Diaphysis

Nutrient canal

☐ cartilage

▨ spongy bone

☐ compact bone

Fig. 14.15 Parts of the growing bone.

The bony structure

Shape
- Is it too wide? (Paget's disease)
- Is it too narrow? (osteogenesis imperfecta)
- Is it bent? (Paget's disease, malunion, rickets)
- Is it fractured?

Density
- Is it increased? (osteopetrosis — marble bones)
- Is it decreased? (osteoporosis, osteomalacia)
- Is it uniform or irregular with loss of normal architecture? (osteomyelitis, fibrous dysplasia)

Periosteum
- Is it visible? (if so, it is abnormal, apart from in infants)
- Is it lifted up, e.g.:
  — callus from a fracture
  — scurvy
  — syphilis

— osteogenic sarcoma

— hypertrophic pulmonary osteoarthropathy

— Caffrey's disease (infantile cortical hyperostosis).

Cortex

- Is it thinner or eroded, e.g. cysts, tumours, aneurysms?
- Is it thicker, e.g. Paget's disease?

Medulla

- Are there any rarefied areas?
- Are these single? e.g.
  — solitary bone cyst
  — Brodie's abscess
  — chondroma
  — giant cell tumour
  — eosinophilic granuloma
  — osteogenic sarcoma (Fig. 14.16)
- Are these multiple? e.g.
  — fibrous dysplasia
  — storage diseases (Gaucher's disease, Hand–Schuller–Christian)
  — sarcoidosis
  — malignant disease
    — secondary carcinoma
    — multiple myeloma
    — leukaemia
- Are there any areas of increased density?
  — single, e.g.
    — aseptic necrosis after trauma
    — septic necrosis (sequestrum)
    — some tumours
  — multiple, e.g.
    — some tumours
    — secondary deposits of prostatic carcinoma
    — Engelmann's disease.

Joints

- The position
  — is it dislocated?
  — is it subluxed?
  — is it in a position of deformity?
- The joint space
  — is it decreased?

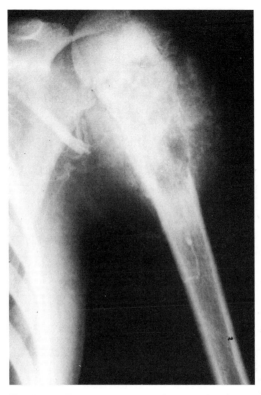

Fig. 14.16 Osteogenic sarcoma of the humerus.

— osteoarthritis (Fig. 14.6)
— rheumatoid arthritis
— is it increased?
— osteochondritis
— Perthe's disease
— distended with fluid
● The joint edge: is there lipping or osteophyte formation?
● The soft tissues
— is there a loose body?
— is there soft tissue calcification, e.g. meniscus?
— is there soft tissue swelling, e.g. bursitis?

Some common contrast techniques

Barium meal
This has now usually been superseded by gastroscopy.

- Barium sulphate in water is the current universal contrast medium for studying the upper gastrointestinal tract.
- Water-soluble-iodine-containing contrast media (e.g. Gastrografin) are of value when a perforation or anastomotic leak is suspected. However, they are contraindicated if there is any danger of pulmonary aspiration. They are also contraindicated in dehydrated infants because of their high osmolarity and hygroscopic characteristics.
- Double contrast techniques utilize air or carbon dioxide to distend the stomach, etc., greatly increasing mucosal definition. Air can be introduced by a nasogastric tube, but more commonly effervescent tablets are used to react with gastric contents to produce carbon dioxide (e.g. sodium bicarbonate, tartaric acid, calcium carbonate).
- Buscopan 20 mg or glucagon 0.1–0.5 mg can be given intravenously to relax the stomach or duodenal wall. Metoclopramide (Maxolon) 20 mg intravenously may increase peristalsis and speed the passage of barium.

Barium enema
- Adequate preliminary bowel preparation is vital — e.g. a low-residue diet for 48 hours, an aperient (e.g. Picolax) 24 hours prior to X-ray, and then possibly regular high-colonic washouts.
- Barium sulphate and water mixture 25% is administered though a rectal catheter by gravity from a height of about 4 feet (1 m 2 cm).
- Double contrast techniques involve introducing air up the catheter once the barium has reached the splenic flexure.
- Colonic spasm can be diminished by intravenous Buscopan 20 mg.

Examination of the biliary tree

Oral cholecystography and intravenous cholangiography
These have been superseded by ultrasound scanning, endoscopic retrograde cholangiopancreatography (ERCP), MRI scanning and percutaneous transhepatic cholangiography (PTC) (see below for scanning techniques).

ERCP
This involves introducing a side-viewing duodenoscope into the second part of the duodenum, and cannulating the ampulla of Vater. This requires a highly skilled endoscopist. Good views can be achieved of both the common bile duct and the pancreatic duct (Fig. 14.17). This procedure may also be used for therapeutic

purposes, for both stone retrieval (Fig. 14.18) and the stenting of malignant strictures (Fig. 14.19). Complications, especially after therapeutic manoeuvres, can include:

- Acute pancreatitis
- Perforation
- Bleeding.

PTC

This involves puncture of the liver percutaneously and identification of a dilated duct (often by ultrasound scanning). Contrast can then be injected into the dilated intrahepatic system and the biliary tree outlined. This approach may also be used therapeutically to insert stents into malignant lesions (Fig. 14.20). Complications can include:

- Bleeding (it is essential to check the clotting screen before PTC)
- Cholangitis
- Biliary peritonitis.

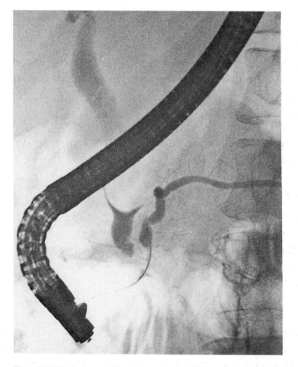

Fig. 14.17 Endoscopic retrograde cholangiopancreatogram (ERCP) showing a large stone in the common bile duct and a normal pancreatic duct.

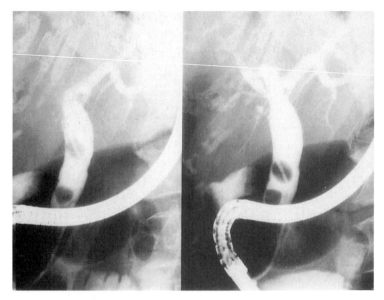

Fig. 14.18 Stone retrieval at ERCP using a balloon catheter.

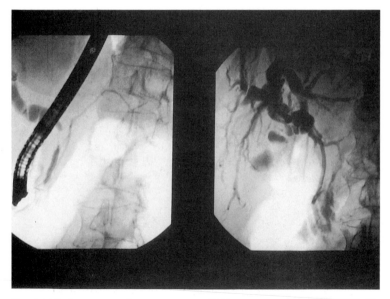

Fig. 14.19 Stenting a malignant stricture at ERCP.

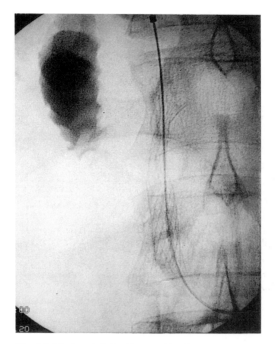

Fig. 14.20 A metal stent inserted by the percutaneous transhepatic route.

Peri-operative cholangiogram (Fig. 14.21)

- Direct cannulation of the common bile duct is undertaken at the time of surgery.
- 25% Hypaque can be injected and films taken after 3 ml, 6 ml and 10 ml of contrast have been used. However, today image intensifiers are in regular use, although it is often important to maintain hard copy as well for medicolegal reasons.
- A normal cholangiogram depends on:
  — normal calibre of duct (maximum 10–12 mm)
  — no filling defects
  — normal intrahepatic tree
  — normal tapering lower end
  — free flow into the duodenum
- The value of post-exploratory 'T'-tube cholangiography is often limited by contrast not passing into the duodenum after the lower duct has been manipulated. The spasm of the sphincter can be diminished by intravenous Buscopan or glucagon.

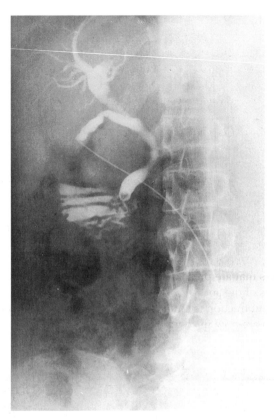

Fig. 14.21 Per-operative cholangiogram showing a stone at the lower end of the common bile duct.

Intravenous urogram
- Patients are fluid restricted, have a plain abdominal film taken, and then receive 20–40 ml of contrast medium intravenously.
- Contrast media used include:
  — Conray (meglumine iothalamate)
  — Hypaque (sodium diatrizoate)
  — Renografin (methylglucamine diatrizoate)
- A compression band just above the symphysis pubis may keep the contrast in the kidneys to allow clearer definition of the upper renal tracts. This should not be used in cases of obstruction, calculi, suspect renal function or aortic aneurysm.
- Films are recorded at 5 and 15 minutes, after compression is released, and up to 2 hours or more if there is an element of hold-up. Tomography may be valuable in delineating renal lesions.

Arteriography

- Contrast media in common use include:
  - Hypaque (sodium diatrizoate)
  - Urografin (mixture of sodium and methylglucamine diatrizoate)
  - Angiografin (meglumine amidotrizoate)
  - Conray (meglumine iothalamate)
  - Triosil (meglumine metrizoate)
  - Renografin (methylglucamine diatrizoate)

  It is obviously not necessary for a candidate to know all these media in detail, but it is advisable to be able to quote details about one specific agent if asked about the technique of arteriography.
- Percutaneous puncture of the femoral artery (Seldinger technique) provides satisfactory distal arteriograms (Fig. 14.22), and selective arterial catheterization can also be achieved using radio-opaque catheters that are preshaped for catheterizing individual branches of the aorta.
- Digital subtraction techniques after either venous or arterial injection are now in common use.

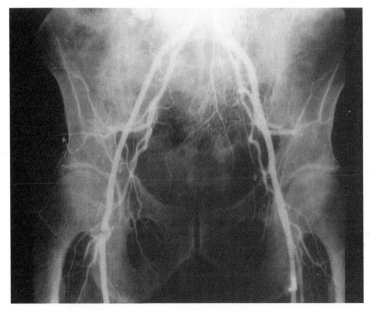

Fig. 14.22 Arteriography showing a stricture at the right-sided bifurcation of the common femoral artery.

- Contrast is injected as quickly as possible and films taken using the automatic changer.
- Translumbar aortography may be performed in certain circumstances under general anaesthetic. It is more hazardous than a Seldinger procedure and is seldom used today, but some claim that it provided better films of the aorta and iliac vessels — although that is disputed, as new catheters and technology mean that excellent quality films can be achieved by free flush within the aorta or by selective catheterization.

Venography (Fig. 14.23)

- Narrow inflatable cuffs are applied to the ankle and knee but not inflated.
- A butterfly needle is inserted into a vein on the foot, which is easier with the foot hanging independently.
- The cuffs are then inflated to obliterate the superficial veins, and up to 50 ml of a low osmolar contrast medium, such as Niopam 300, are injected.
- Screening is undertaken while injecting, with neutral and internal and external rotational views. Good views should be obtained of the deep veins and any incompetent perforators.

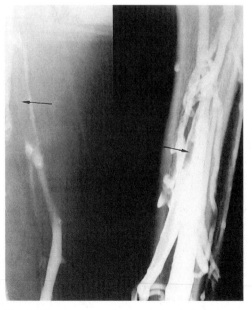

Fig. 14.23 Venogram showing deep vein thrombosis.

Lymphangiography

- 0.5 ml of 2.5% patent blue violet dye is injected subcutaneously into the toe webs. The dye is then taken up by the lymphatic channels.
- Under local anaesthetic, a transverse incision on the dorsum of the foot is used to expose a suitable lymphatic vessel.
- A needle is introduced into the vessel, saline injected, and, if there is no leak, the needle is secured in site by a catgut ligature.
- If the lymphangiogram is being done to investigate primary lymphoedema, a water-soluble contrast medium like Conray 280 should be used. However, for examination of the lymph vessels and nodes, an oily medium is commonly used, such as ultrafluid lipiodol. This is administered at 7 ml/h using a pump, up to a maximum of 10 ml per limb.
- The first films are taken as soon as the contrast is all in, and at 24 hours and 48 hours to assess the proximal flow and pattern of uptake by the lymph nodes.

Some common scanning techniques

Ultrasound scanning

Principles
- Depends upon the varying ability of body tissues to absorb sound.
- When an ultrasonic wave strikes a tissue interface, each with a differing acoustic impedance, some of the energy is reflected (Fig. 14.24) and can be detected by a detector in line with the generating ultrasonic beam.
- The echo can be displayed on an oscilloscope as an undimensional wave (A scan) or if a sweeping beam is used, a two-dimensional black and white picture can be constructed (B scan).
- The intensity of the image can reflect the amplitude of the reflected wave and produce a picture of varying shades of grey (grey-scale ultrasound).
- Ultrasound is non-invasive and carries no radiation risk and is therefore safe.
- It has high resolution and can be used to monitor the progression of certain pathological processes, e.g. pancreatic cysts.
- Ultrasound scanning can be used to direct biopsy needles.
- Intraoperative or endoluminal scanning can be used, e.g. endoanal, endoscopic.
- Ultrasonic flow meters function on the Doppler principle, utilizing the movement of red cells to cause a shift in the frequency of the reflected signal.

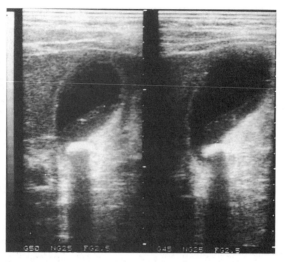

Fig. 14.24 Ultrasound of the gall bladder showing an obvious stone in the neck of the gall bladder with an acoustic shadow behind it.

- Duplex scanning is achieved by using pulsed or continuous-wave Doppler and colour mapping with the two-dimensional images produced by B mode scanning.

Computerized tomography scanning (CT)

Principles
- The patient is placed in centre of scanner and X-ray tube rotates around him/her.
- A computer integrates the multiple X-ray projections to produce an image.
- Images are usually reconstructed in axial plane (Fig. 14.25).
- More recent helical/spiral CT scanning involves the patient moving through the gantry while the X-ray tube rotates continuously following a helical path.
- A CT image is a matrix of pixels each having a grey-scale representing the X-ray attenuation value of the tissues, e.g.:
  — fat and gas have negative attenuation values and are black
  — bone has a high attenuation value and is white
  — intravenous contrast medium can artificially increase local attenuation (Fig. 14.26).
- A high dose of irradiation is required and where possible should be avoided in younger patients and women of childbearing age.
- Artefacts produced by barium, metallic clips, stents, etc.

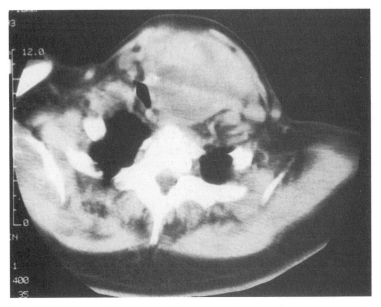

Fig. 14.25 CT scan of the neck and chest showing tracheal compression and deviation by a large goitre.

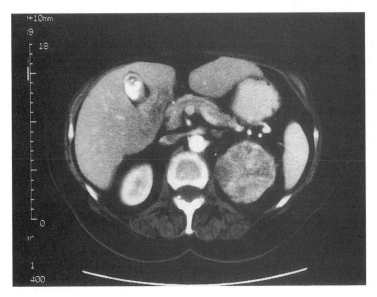

Fig. 14.26 CT scan with contrast showing a left renal tumour and gallstones. Also note that the pancreatic duct can be clearly seen.

Magnetic resonance image scanning (MRI)

Principles

- The patient is placed in a powerful magnetic field with which all the protons in the body become aligned.
- Radio waves transmitted into the patient cause the alignment of the protons to change.
- When the radiofrequency pulse is turned off the protons return to their neutral position, emitting their own radiowave signals which are picked up by a receiver coil.
- These signals are used to generate an image which depends not only on the proton density but on the way the protons resonate in their local environment.
- The image comprises an array of pixels, as in CT scanning, but there is greater contrast resolution with MRI than with CT (Fig. 14.27).
- The natural contrast of MRI can be increased with contrast agents such as intravenous chelated gadolinium compounds, e.g. Gd-DTPA.
- MRI avoids the use of ionizing radiation and is therefore safe.
- MRI should be avoided in any patients with metal clips, stents, pacemakers.

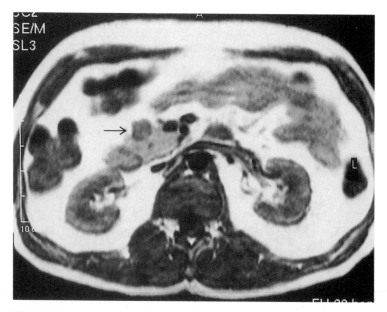

Fig. 14.27 MRI scan demonstrating a mass in the head of the pancreas that was in fact a gastrinoma (arrowed).

Radionuclide scanning

Principles
- Radionuclide imaging is based on a form of autoemission, a quantity of radioactive material being administered to the patient.
- The radioactivity is administered as radiopharmaceutical agent that is chosen so that it follows a specific metabolic pathway, e.g. radio-iodine and thyroid uptake.
- Images can demonstrate the outline of an organ, with a potential to assess the extent to which it is functioning by means of indicating areas of abnormally low uptake or abnormally high uptake (Fig. 14.28).

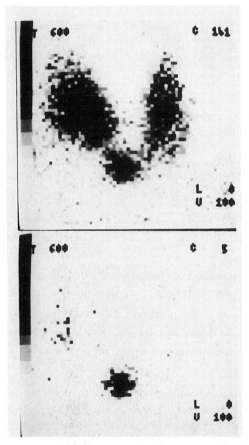

Fig. 14.28 Radionuclide thallium/technetium subtraction scan showing residual activity representing a parathyroid adenoma.

- Imaging depends upon the measurement of γ-photons from sites of radioactivity. To do this a gamma camera is utilized, with four fundamental processes:
  — collimation (a multichannelling device to allow spatial resolution)
  — scintillation detection
  — electronic signal processing
  — display of information.

Examples of radionuclides

Liver
- ^{99m}Tc-labelled sulphur colloid for reticuloendothelial scanning
- ^{75}Se-labelled methionine in liver cell tumours
- ^{67}Ga citrate for liver abscesses or tumour location
- ^{111}Indium-labelled white blood cells for foci of infection
- ^{99m}Tc-labelled butyl-imino-diacetic acid (BIDA) for excretion.

Small bowel
- ^{99m}Tc pertechnetate for Meckel's diverticulum (Fig. 14.29)
- ^{51}Cr-labelled red blood cells for assessing blood loss
- ^{57}Co-labelled vitamin B_{12} for the Schilling test.

Thyroid
- ^{131}I to search for metastases from differentiated thyroid carcinoma and for therapy.

Parathyroid (Fig. 14.28)
- ^{201}Tl thallous chloride/^{99m}Tc pertechnetate subtraction scan.

Adrenal glands
- ^{75}Se 6-selenomethylnorcholesterol for the cortex
- ^{123}I or ^{131}I meta-iodobenzylguanidine (m-IBG) for the medulla.

Kidneys
- ^{99m}Tc-labelled diethylene-triaminepenta-acetate (DTPA)
- ^{99m}Tc-labelled dimercaptosuccinic acid (DMSA).

Lungs
- Ventilation/perfusion scanning for pulmonary embolism
- ^{99m}Tc-labelled microaggregates of albumin for perfusion
- ^{81m}Kr gas for ventilation studies (xenon can be used).

Bone
- ^{99m}Tc-labelled hydroxymethylene diphosphonate (HDP).

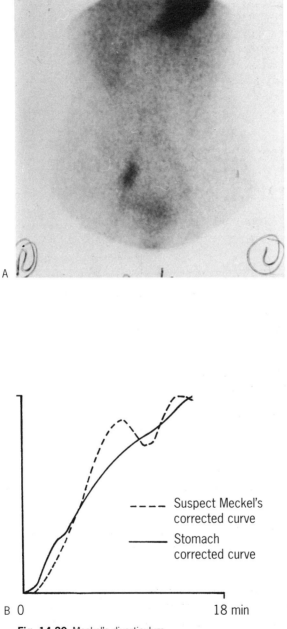

Fig. 14.29 Meckel's diverticulum.
A. Positive technetium scan for a Meckel's diverticulum.
B. The uptake of the Meckel's diverticulum compared with the stomach uptake.

Clinical pathology with principles of surgery

15

During this viva clinically related pathology topics will be discussed, and any principles relating to the practice of surgery in general. The first 10 minutes will be with a pathologist, who will cover topics such as clinical pathology, haematology, microbiology and biochemistry. The second 10 minutes will be with a surgeon, who will review a candidate's question subject sheet from the rest of the examination and will seek to ensure that the syllabus has been covered with no repetition.

Because of the nature of the content of this viva it is not possible to predict so easily the topics that may be asked. However, remember that the examiners may again have X-rays, instruments, bones, clinical photographs, etc., with which to start a discussion. The following topics may help to formulate answers and stimulate further reading relevant to this viva.

Some useful definitions

Inflammation	The response of living tissue to injury
Tumour	An abnormal mass of tissue, the growth of which exceeds and is uncoordinated with that of the normal tissues, and persists in the same excessive manner after cessation of the stimuli which evoked the change (after Willis)
Hamartoma	An abnormal tumour-like malformation in which the tissues of a particular part of the body are arranged in an haphazard fashion, often with an excess of one or more of its components
Ulcer	An abnormal break in an epithelial surface
Fistula	An abnormal communication between two epithelial surfaces
Sinus	An abnormal blind ending tract opening onto an epithelial surface

Hernia	An abnormal protrusion of a viscus or part of a viscus through an opening. (The opening itself may be normal — e.g. the femoral canal — or abnormal — e.g. an incisional hernia)
Teratoma	A tumour composed of a variety of tissues, usually containing representatives of the three primitive germ cell layers, and in a situation where these tissues do not normally occur
Atrophy	A reduction in size of individual cells leading to a diminution in size and function of an organ. This is usually due to lack of use or nutrition, and is an acquired condition
Agenesis	Complete failure of development of an organ or part of an organ
Hypoplasia	Failure of development of an organ to full mature size
Aplasia	Occasionally used to describe severe hypoplasia. Now a haematological term for marrow damage leading to pancytopaenia
Hypertrophy	The increase in size of an organ due to an increase in size of its individual cells, e.g. cardiac left ventricular hypertrophy in systemic hypertension
Hyperplasia	The increase in size of an organ due to an increase in the number of its cells, e.g. primary thyrotoxicosis
Metaplasia	A change in type of differentiation from one form of tissue to another similarly, but usually less specialized, differentiated tissue — e.g. squamous metaplasia in the gall bladder, renal pelvis, bladder, uterus or bronchus
Dysplasia	Disordered cellular development. May accompany hyperplasia and metaplasia, and is characterized by increased mitosis, irregular nuclei and a disordered cellular arrangement. The term is often confusing as in certain cases it is associated with premaligant conditions — the cervix, stomach, colon etc. — while in other conditions there is no suggestion of incipient neoplastic change — e.g. fibrous dysplasia of bone, mammary dysplasia
Dyscrasia	Literally means 'bad mixture'. Now is used only by haematologists to describe blood disorders of uncertain origin.

The pathological (surgical) sieve

Congenital

Congenital

- Those developing during foetal life, e.g.:
  — anal atresia
  — tracheo-oesophageal fistula
- Those acquired during foetal life, e.g. rubella or syphilis infection causing foetal abnormalities.

Genetically determined

- Those apparent at birth, e.g. Down syndrome with its associated abnormalities of facial, cardiac and skeletal defects
- Those developing in adolescence or adult life, e.g. polyposis coli (Fig. 15.1).

Acquired

Physical agents

- Direct trauma, e.g. stabbing, gun shots, fractures
- Heat, e.g. burns, scalds
- Cold, e.g. frostbite, trench foot
- Ultraviolet light
- Electricity
- Irradiation, e.g. burns, contractures, telangiectasia, strictures.

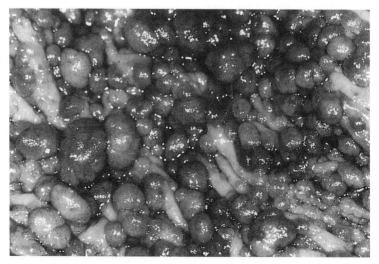

Fig. 15.1 Polyposis coli.

Chemicals

- Organic or inorganic
- Smoking, e.g.:
  — peripheral vascular disease
  — pulmonary disease
- Drugs, e.g.:
  — enteric potassium causing jejunoileal ulceration (Fig. 15.2)
  — phenacitin causing renal papillary necrosis
- Alcohol, e.g.:
  — cirrhosis
  — acute and chronic pancreatitis
- Chemicals
  — those with a general effect on cells, e.g. cyanide
  — those that cause local injury associated with acute inflammation, e.g. strong acids and alkalis
  — those with more or less selective injury to particular organs or cell types, e.g.:
    — alcohol and hepatocyte damage leading to cirrhosis
    — arsenic and squamous cell carcinoma of the skin
    — asbestos and lung cancer
    — aniline dye and rubber workers and transitional cell carcinoma of the bladder: the chemicals involved being:
      — β-naphthylamine
      — benzidine
      — xenylamine.

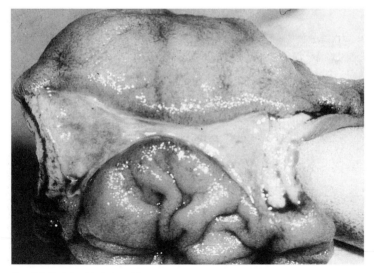

Fig. 15.2 Jejunoileal ulceration.

Inflammation

- Non-specific:
  - acute, e.g. acute appendicitis
  - subacute, e.g. subacute salpingitis
  - chronic, e.g. chronic cholecystitis
- Specific:
  - acute, e.g. actinomycosis
  - chronic, e.g.:
    - tuberculosis
    - syphilis
    - leprosy
- Infections
  - bacterial
  - viral
  - rickettsial
  - fungal
  - protozoal
  - metazoal.

Immunological

- Hypersensitivity, e.g.:
  - anaphylaxis
  - asthma
- Autoimmunity, e.g.:
  - thyroiditis
  - systemic lupus.

Ischaemia, leading to:

- Atrophy, e.g. cerebral atrophy
- Infarction, e.g. myocardial infarction
- Gangrene, e.g.:
  - peripheral vascular disease (Fig. 9.2)
  - strangulated gut (Fig. 15.3).

Mechanical

Obstruction of any lumen, e.g.:
- Gut
  - outside the gut
    - herniae
    - band (Fig. 15.4)
    - adhesions
    - volvulus (Fig. 15.5)
  - in the wall

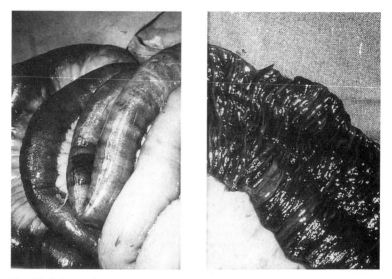

Fig. 15.3 Strangulated ischaemic small bowel from within large femoral hernia.

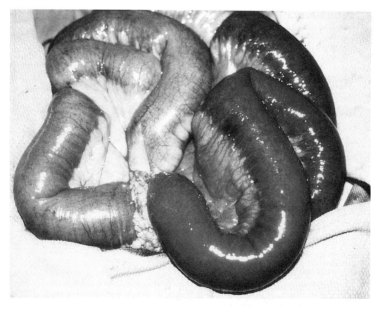

Fig. 15.4 Band obstruction of small bowel.

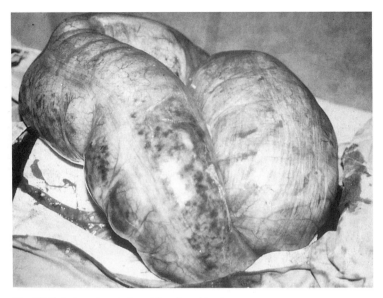

Fig. 15.5 Ischaemic volvulus of the sigmoid colon.

- — tumours
- — strictures
- — intussusception (Fig. 15.6)
- — in the lumen
  - — foreign body
  - — food bolus
  - — gallstone ileus (Fig. 15.7)
- Lung
  - — obstructive pulmonary collapse
  - — inhaled foreign body
  - — mucus
  - — tumour
- Kidney
  - — hydronephrosis
  - — tumour
  - — calculi
  - — reflux.

Metabolic

- Deficiencies, e.g.:
  - — iodine causing endemic goitre and cretinism
  - — vitamin deficiencies, e.g. beri-beri
- Intrinsic metabolic abnormalities, e.g. gout

A

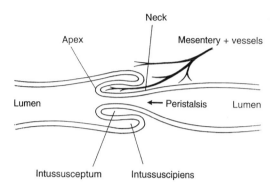

B

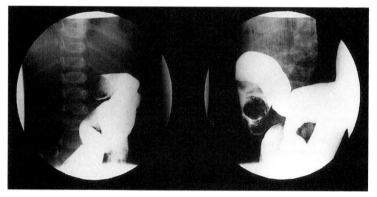

Fig. 15.6 Intussusception
A. Diagrammatic representation of an intussusception.
B. Barium enema of a child with intussusception showing partial hydrostatic reduction.

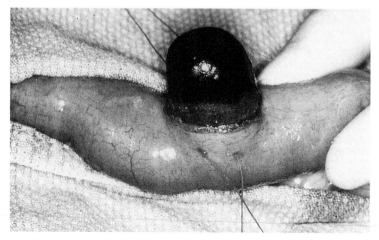

Fig. 15.7 Gallstone ileus.

Endocrine disorders

- Hypofunction, e.g.:
  - diabetes mellitus
  - myxoedema
  - Addison's disease
- Hyperfunction
  - thyrotoxicosis
  - Cushing's disease
  - hyperparathyroidism.

Degenerations

- Fatty change in the liver
- Hyaline degeneration
- Mucoid degeneration, e.g. medionecrosis of the aorta.

Infiltrations

- Amyloid
- Glycogen in heart and kidney in diabetes mellitus
- Other glycogen storage diseases.

Neoplasia

- Benign
- Malignant
  - primary
  - secondary.

Neoplasia according to 'tissue of origin'

Epithelium
- Benign
  - surface epithelium: papilloma (Fig. 15.8)
  - glandular epithelium: adenoma (Fig. 15.9)
- Malignant: carcinoma
  - squamous cell
  - transitional cell
  - adenocarcinoma (Fig. 15.10)
    - papillary
    - cystadenocarcinoma
    - spheroidal cell
    - clear cell.

Connective tissue
- Benign, e.g.
  - lipoma (Fig. 7.1)

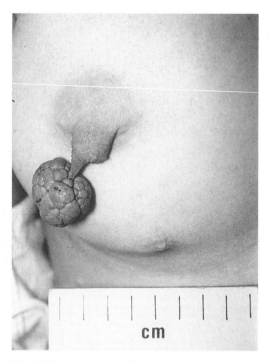

Fig. 15.8 Benign skin papilloma of the nipple.

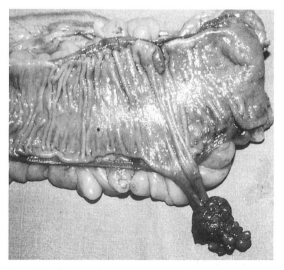

Fig. 15.9 Benign adenomatous polyp of the colon.

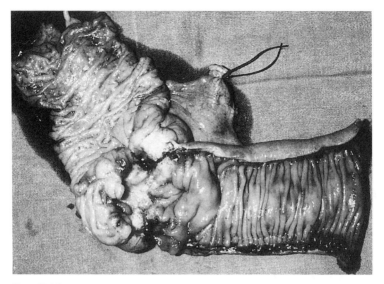

Fig. 15.10 Adenocarcinoma of the caecum.

— fibroma
— leiomyoma
— chondroma
— osteoma
— myxoma
● Malignant, e.g. sarcoma (many varieties).

Lymphoid tissue
● Malignant, e.g.:
— Hodgkin's disease
— non-Hodgkin's lymphoma.

Naevus cells
● Benign, e.g. benign naevus
● Malignant, e.g. malignant melanoma (Fig. 7.3).

Nervous system (dependent on cell of origin)
● Nerve cell: neuroblastoma
● Glial cell
— glioma
— astrocytoma
— oligodendroglioma
— ependymoma
● Meninges: meningioma
● Medulloblast: medulloblastoma

- Microglia
    - microglioma
    - (lymphoma)
- Nerve sheath: schwannoma.

Endothelium
- Benign, e.g.
    - haemangioma
    - lymphangioma
- Malignant, e.g. haemangioendothelioma.

Embryonic tissue
- Benign, e.g.:
    - benign teratoma
    - ovarian dermoid
- Malignant, e.g.
    - malignant teratoma (Fig. 15.11)
    - nephroblastoma
    - hepatoblastoma

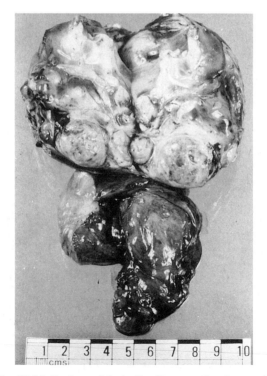

Fig. 15.11 Teratoma of the testis with very oedematous cord.

Many tumours are intermediate or inconsistent in their behavioural characteristics and are difficult to classify as either benign or malignant.

Intermediate tumours
Examples include:

- Basal cell carcinoma
- Some salivary gland tumours like pleomorphic adenomas
- Carcinoid tumours
- Giant cell tumours of bone
- Many gliomas
- Ameloblastoma
- Craniopharyngioma.

Hamartomas
See page 189 for definition. Example: hamartoma of the lung.
Most haemangiomata are in fact hamartomas rather than true tumours.

Miscellaneous
- Idiopathic: cause not known (cryptogenic), e.g. ulcerative colitis (Fig. 15.12)
- Iatrogenic: induced by a physician (even occasionally by a surgeon!)
- Psychogenic.

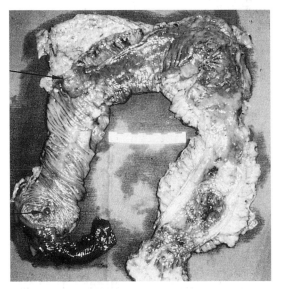

Fig. 15.12 Ulcerative colitis showing almost total colitis but with caecal sparing (note the arrowed polypoid carcinoma of transverse colon and the caecal polyp).

Neoplasia

For each neoplastic lesion consider the following characteristics:

- Incidence
- Appearance
- Staging
- Grading
- Patterns of behaviour
- Spread
- Tumour effects
  — local
  — general
- Carcinogenesis
- Prognosis
- Survival.

Incidence

For the incidence of deaths from malignant disease in England and Wales, see Table 15.1.

Table 15.1 – Deaths from malignant disease in England and Wales

Oesophagus	5 800	Small bowel	200
Stomach	7 000	Colon	10 800
Liver (primary)	600	Rectum	5 000
Lung	32 000	Pancreas	5 800
Breast	12 000	Malignant melanoma	1 400
Testis	100	Prostate	8 900
Bladder	4 800	Ovary	3 900
Leukaemia	3 500	Kidney	2 600
Lymphoma	4 000		
All neoplasms	141 300		
Road traffic accidents	3 000		
Myocardial infarction	134 000		

*approximate figures

Tumour appearance

- Annular: likely to obstruct lumen
- Fungating: likely to bleed and ulcerate
- Scirrhous: discrete and firm
- Encephaloid: soft and more diffuse.

Tumour staging

E.g. breast carcinoma TNM staging

T: primary tumour

- T0: no demonstrable tumour
- T1: less than 2 cm
  — T1a: with no fixation to fascia or muscle
  — T1b: with fixation to underlying fascia and/or muscle
- T2: more than 2 cm, but less than 5 cm
  — T2a: with no fixation to fascia or muscle
  — T2b: with fixation to underlying fascia and/or muscle
- T3: more than 5 cm
  — T3a: with no fixation to fascia or muscle
  — T3b: with fixation to underlying fascia and/or muscle

(Note: skin dimpling and nipple retraction can occur in T1, T2, or T3 lesions)

- T4: of any size with direct extension to chest wall or skin (i.e. ribs, intercostal muscles and serratus anterior, but not pectoral muscle)
  — T4a: with fixation to chest wall
  — T4b: with oedema, ulceration of skin, peau d'orange or satellite skin nodules
  — T4c: both of above.

N: regional lymph nodes
- N0: no palpable axillary nodes
- N1: movable homolateral axillary nodes
  — N1a: not considered to contain tumour
  — N1b: considered to contain tumour
- N2: fixed homolateral axillary nodes
- N3: supraclavicular or infraclavicular nodes or oedema of the arm.

M: distant metastases
— M0: no evidence of metastases
— M1: distant metastases present.

Stage grouping

Stage I	T1	N0, N1a	M0
Stage II	T0	N1b	
	T1	N1b	M0
	T2	N0, N1a, N1b	

Stage III	T3	Any N	
	T4	Any N	M0
	Any T	N2, N3	
Stage IV	Any T	Any N	M1

Modified Duke's classification for colorectal carcinoma
Grade A: confined to the wall
Grade B: extended through the wall
Grade C1: involvement of pararectal nodes
Grade C2: involvement of distal nodes, such as preaortic nodes
Grade D: distal metastases.

Grading of tumours
E.g. Broder's classification (infrequently used now)

I 25% of lesion undifferentiated
II 25–50% of lesion undifferentiated
III 50–75% of lesion undifferentiated
IV Over 75% of lesion undifferentiated (anaplastic).

Patterns of behaviour
- Intermediate, e.g. basal cell carcinoma
- Latent carcinoma, e.g. prostatic carcinoma in elderly men
- Carcinoma in situ, e.g. cervix (preinvasive proliferation)
- Spontaneous regression, e.g.:
  — malignant melanoma
  — renal cell carcinoma
  — neuroblastoma
  — choriocarcinoma
- Dormant carcinoma, e.g. late appearance of secondary deposits in breast carcinoma.

Patterns of metastatic spread
- Local invasion: all malignant tumours
- Lymphatic, e.g. carcinoma of the breast
- Blood, e.g.:
  — to lungs, liver, brain, etc.
  — to bone
    — osteolytic, e.g. kidney
    — osteosclerotic, e.g. prostate
    — others: lung, breast, thyroid
- Transcoelomic, e.g. peritoneal seedlings from carcinoma of colon, stomach, etc.

Effects of tumour presence

General
- Malaise
- Cachexia
- Weight loss
- Anaemia.

Local effects from the primary tumour itself
- Intestinal obstruction
- Bleeding
- Pain from
  — pressure
  — nerve involvement
  — obstruction of viscus
- Palpable mass
- Individual specific/systemic effects, e.g.:
  — renal cell carcinoma
    — pyrexia
    — polycythaemia
    — hypertension
    — haematuria
  — bronchogenic carcinoma
    — endocrine effects
    — neurological effects
    — encephalopathy
    — myelopathy
    — peripheral neuropathy

Secondary effects from metastases
- Pathological fractures
- Jaundice (liver deposits)
- Anaemia (marrow involvement)
- Neurological disorders, e.g.:
  — spinal deposits
  — cerebral deposits
- dyspnoea, e.g. lung deposits.

Carcinogenesis

Physical agents
- Sunlight: squamous or basal cell carcinoma
- Burns: clay pipe smokers and lip carcinoma
- Marjolin's ulcer in scars of old burns, sinuses, ulcers, etc.
- Leukoplakia, e.g. tongue, vulva.

Chemicals
- Skin carcinoma
  — coal tar derivatives
  — shale oil
  — arsenic
- Lung carcinoma
  — smoking
  — asbestos
  — nickel workers
  — chromium workers
  — haematite workers
- Bladder carcinoma
  — aniline dye workers
  — rubber workers.

Irradiation
- Skin carcinoma
- Leukaemia
- Lung carcinoma (e.g. in the Schneeberg and Joachimsthal miners exposed to radon).

Hormones
- Breast carcinoma (oestrogen status)
- Uterine carcinoma.

Nutritional
Post-cricoid carcinoma in iron deficiency.

Chronic irritation
Leading to metaplasia and dysplasia, e.g.:

- Schistosomiasis in bladder cancer
- Long-standing ulcerative colitis (Fig. 15.12)
- Post-gastrectomy stump cancer.

Factors affecting prognosis
- Anatomical site (the specific size of a tumour can either lead to early detection or cause fatal complications)
- Histology and grading
- Clinical staging
- Intercurrent disease
- Tumour to host relationship.

Survival rates
Survival rates depend upon various factors, as shown below.

Staging (e.g. breast and colorectal cancer)
Average 5-year survival rates:

Breast (stage)		Colorectal cancer (Dukes)	
I	84%	A	92%
II	71%	B	71%
III	48%	C1	40%
IV	18%	C2	27%
		D	16%

Differentiation (e.g. thyroid)
Average 5-year survival rates:

Anaplastic	0%
Well-differentiated	90%

Local depth (extent) (e.g. malignant melanoma)
Average 10-year survival rates (with no nodal or distant metastases):

Depth of spread	< 1mm	95%
	1–4 mm	70%
	> 4 mm	40%

Resectability (e.g. lung)
Average 5-year survival rates:

Resectable	30%
Irresectable	0%

Geographical location (e.g. stomach)
Average 5-year survival rates:

Europe	10%
USA	15%
Japan	30%

Non-surgical treatment of malignancy

The principles of management of malignant disease need to be clearly
understood. In most cases surgery remains the mainstay of therapy,
especially for the control or removal of the primary tumour. However,
other modalities of treatment are playing an increasingly important
role in the management of malignancy, both as primary treatment

and as adjuvant therapy or for palliative control of symptoms. The basic principles of these different modalities of treatment need to be understood, along with their advantages and limitations.

Radiotherapy

Principles of action
- When X-rays pass through the nucleus of a cell they can directly or indirectly alter the structure of DNA, resulting in cell death. A cell is most vulnerable to the effects of irradiation during mitosis and least vulnerable during the 'S' phase of DNA replication (Fig. 15.13).
- Irradiation has most effect on rapidly dividing tissues.
- Radiotherapy is less effective in hypoxic tissues.
- Fractionated radiotherapy, in which smaller doses are given intermittently rather than the same total dose at one sitting, allows more selective treatment which takes into consideration the speed of reaction to radiotherapy of tissues and tumour and allows an intervening period for repair of sublethal damage of other tissues.

Methods of administration

External beam
This uses X-rays from a linear accelerator or gamma rays from a cobalt teletherapy unit

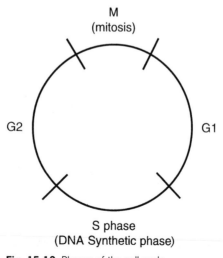

Fig. 15.13 Phases of the cell cycle.

Intracavitary
Short-distance radiotherapy (brachytherapy) involves placing radio-active sources such as caesium or radium into natural cavities, for example the uterus. 'Afterloading' — i.e. activation of radioactivity remotely so as not to expose staff to irradiation — has made this method of management safer.

Interstitial
This is another from of brachytherapy in which radioactive wires, needles or seeds of iridium or ^{125}I are directly inserted into tumour tissue — e.g. breast cancer, head and neck cancers, soft tissue sarcomas.

Ingestion
This utilizes tumour specificity of uptake of a radioactive compound and is exemplified by radioiodine use for well-differentiated thyroid carcinoma. Tracer doses of radioiodine can be used to assess any residual thyroid tissue, followed by an ablative dose. Following ablation sequential scans and/or thyroglobulin levels can be used as markers for any recurrent disease, which may indicate the need for a further therapeutic dose of radioiodine.

Chemotherapy
There are four main groups of cytotoxic agents:

Alkylating agents
E.g. cyclophosphamide, melphalan, busulphan, cis-platinum, nitrosoureas. Act by forming covalent bonds with bases in DNA (e.g. guanine) and preventing normal replication, leading to cell death. Alkylating agents vary in their anti-tumour activity and toxicity.

Antimetabolites
E.g. methotrexate, 5-fluorouracil, 6-mercaptopurine, hydroxyurea. Act by being mistaken for normal DNA substrates and thus disrupting the cell during 'S' phase (Fig. 15.13).

Antibiotics
E.g. actinomycin D, adriamycin (doxorubicin), bleomycin, mitomycin C. Act by various differing mechanisms producing single-strand breaks in DNA analogous to the effect of irradiation.

Alkaloids
E.g. vincristine, vinblastine. Act by destroying the mitotic spindle by binding to tubulin.

Clinical use of cytotoxic agents

For any clinical usage of such an agent the oncologist needs to consider the following:

- Is the clinical indication for:
  — a potential cure (e.g. lymphomas)?
  — effective palliation (e.g. breast, colorectal)?
- What is a safe dose range?
- What is the most appropriate route of administration?
- What is an agent's potential toxicity?
- What is an agent's route of elimination?
- Is there any overlap of toxicity in agents used in combination therapy?

Combination therapy

Drug combination

- Allows maximal impact on cell destruction with minimal overlap of toxicity of cytotoxic agents
- Provides a broader range of activity against cells in a heterogenous tumour
- Slows any development of new resistant cell lines.

Therapy combination

Surgery, radiotherapy and chemotherapy may be combined depending on the tumour under consideration, e.g.:

- Irradiation of a tumour bed after tumour excision
- Certain agents (e.g. 5-FU, cis-platinum) may sensitize cells to irradiation

Hormonal therapy

This relates to tumours that are 'hormone-responsive', such as breast and prostate.

Agents

- Anti-oestrogens, e.g. tamoxifen
- Progestins, e.g. megestrol acetate
- Aromatase inhibitors, e.g. aminoglutethimide
- Luteinizing hormone releasing hormone agonists, e.g. Zoladex.

These agents have now rendered such ablative operative procedures as adrenalectomy, hypophysectomy and orchidectomy virtually obsolete.

Immunotherapy

The use of immunotherapy in many cases is still undergoing active research. The use of monoclonal antibodies is still experimental and thus far has not lived up to the dramatic expectations initially promised. The use of compounds such as interleukin has not yet produced consistent results but BCG (Bacille Calmette-Guérin) is in current use. This has been found to be active in bladder cancer as it appears to have both a direct toxic action on the transitional epithelium and an immunological effect by stimulating a mononuclear infiltrate. This in turn may have both a specific and a non-specific immune effect on the elimination of tumour cells.

Mechanical

These methods tend to be palliative, with particular reference to avoiding obstructive-type symptoms; for example:

- Intubation, e.g. oesophageal carcinoma (Atkinson, Celestin)
- Stenting, e.g.:
  — biliary and pancreatic malignancy
    — endoscopic stenting (at ERCP)
    — transhepatic (radiologically screened) (metal or plastic)
  — ureteric: double 'J' stents
- Debulking tumour, e.g. oesophageal, gastric, rectal tumours
  — laser
  — diathermy fulguration.

Inflammation

The following may well be discussion points:

The cardinal signs of inflammation

- Calor: heat
- Rubor: redness
- Dolor: pain
- Tumor: swelling

Celsus described these four features in the first century. A fifth has since been added and attributed to either Galen or John Hunter without grounds of verification:

- Functio laesa: loss of function.

Macroscopical variants of acute inflammation

- Serous, e.g. pleural effusion

- Fibrinous, e.g. peritonitis
- Haemorrhagic, e.g. pancreatitis
- Suppurative, e.g. abscess, empyema
- Catarrhal, e.g. respiratory tract infection
- Gangrenous, e.g. acute gangrenous appendicitis, clostridial infections
- Phlegmonous, e.g. spreading infections of the neck
- Cellulitis, e.g. spreading red-raised inflammation usually due to β-haemolytic streptococci
- Membranous, e.g.:
  — usually false membrane
  — diphtheria
  — pseudomembranous colitis.

Forms of necrosis

- Coagulative necrosis, e.g. myocardial infarction
- Colliquative necrosis, e.g. cerebral infarction
- Caseation necrosis, e.g. tuberculous lesion
- Fat necrosis
  — traumatic, e.g. breast
  — enzymic, e.g. pancreatitis
- Suppurative, e.g. acute gangrenous appendicitis
- Fibrinoid necrosis, e.g.:
  — connective tissue disorders
  — rheumatic fever
  — rheumatoid arthritis
- Gummatous necrosis, e.g. the necrosis of tertiary syphilis
- Gangrene: tissue necrosis in bulk, usually with superimposed putrefaction.

Transplantation

Type of graft
- Autograft: transplant in same individual (autogenous graft)
- Isograft: transplant with identical genotype, i.e. identical twins (syngeneic graft)
- Allograft: transplant between members of same species (homograft)
- Xenograft: transplant between members of different species (heterograft)
- Structural graft: to act as a non-living scaffold, e.g.:
  — heart valves
  — vascular prosthesis.

Position of graft
- Orthotopic: transplant to anatomically normal site
- Heterotopic: transplant to anatomically abnormal site.

Method of grafting
- Free graft, e.g. skin graft
- Vascularized graft, e.g. kidney, liver
- Pedicle graft, i.e. initially remains attached to donor site.

Frequency of grafting
- First set: initial transplant
- Second set: second and subsequent grafts.

Tissue typing
- ABO blood groups
- Lymphocyte histocompatibility tests
- HLA system
- Major histocompatibility locus complex (MHC).

Immunosuppression
- Steroids
- Azathioprine
- Anti-lymphocytic globulin
- Cyclosporin A.

Organs
- Kidney
- Liver
- Pancreas
- Small bowel
- Heart (heart and lungs)
- Bone marrow.

Donors
- Live donors
  — identical twins
  — related donor
  — non-related donor
- Cadaver donor.

Stoma management

In any discussion regarding stomas the following factors may need to be considered:

Forms

- Temporary loop defunctioning colostomy
- Temporary loop ileostomy
- Ileostomy (spout — Brooke)
- Continent ileostomy (Kock)
- Permanent end colostomy
- Mucous fistula
- Paul-Mikulicz procedure
- Hartmann's procedure
- Caecostomies are not to be encouraged.

Practical considerations

- Siting
- Appliances
- Control of effluent (including irrigation technique)
- Complications
  - recession
  - obstruction
  - prolapse
  - fistula
  - skin excoriation
  - herniation.

Final hints on examination technique

16

General comments

Remember this is basically a clinical examination, and the examiner is looking to see whether you possess the necessary qualities both to be a Member or Associate Fellow of the Royal College of Surgeons and to enter the phase of higher surgical training. Therefore your manner with the patients and your courtesy and compassion are just as important facets and features of your clinical practice as is your clinical knowledge.

You should aim to come across as a knowledgeable, reliable and organized individual without giving the impression of being 'cocky' or a 'know-all'. You should appear interested in the clinical practice of surgery and give the impression that you can be trusted with the everyday management of sick patients.

So many candidates fail themselves either by being inadequately prepared or by saying something stupid in the 'heat of the moment' while under pressure. It is disappointing enough to fail any examination through an unfortunate but significant gap in one's knowledge, but it is tragic to fail through stupidity. This book has sought to advise on your preparation and to help you 'think before you leap'. Take every opportunity to practise examining short cases under pressure and to improve your viva technique. Make sure that you are adequately prepared before you sit each section of the examination. It is a false economy of time to take any section too early and fail it. This merely wastes money and discourages you. Endeavour to prepare well, with respect to both clinical experience and academic knowledge, and then sit the examination when you feel that you are likely to pass each section at your first go. If you have completed good clinical jobs and assiduously followed a distance learning course such as the STEP course published by the Royal College of Surgeons of England, there is every chance that you will indeed pass at your first attempt.

Dos and Don'ts in examination technique

Do...

- Be courteous.
- Dress neatly and sit up smartly in the chair. It does not create a good impression if you are too casually dressed, and sit cross-legged, rocking back in your chair with your hands in your pockets (Fig. 16.1).
- Demonstrate the right degree of humility, without being obsequious or 'greasy'. Examiners can easily see through 'bullshitters'.
- Be honest. The experienced examiner can easily see through candidates who claim to have experience that they do not possess. Once you are caught out being dishonest, all is lost.
- Speak up but don't shout or speak too loudly as there are other candidates in the room. You need to sound authoritative and yet not overconfident. This comes with practice.
- Accurately answer the question. Try to give a well-formulated answer to the exact question you have been asked. This will again only come by practice, and can be achieved most easily by using headings and classifications.
- Think clinical. Try to give answers and treatment recommendations that would be practical and appropriate in your own clinical setting. Don't be panicked into saying something different just because this is an examination.

Don't...

- Guess.
- Lie.
- Argue — even if you think you are right! Remember that in an examination 'the examiner is always right'. However, you are entitled to hold your own opinion, but only as long as that opinion can be backed up by references or by legitimate experience. This is particularly true for the Operative Surgery viva. All surgeons have their own preferred technique for an operation, but 'there is more than one way to skin a cat'. Personal prejudice is inevitable but most examiners will accept an alternative method to their own, as long as it is a recognized method, and you can substantiate its advantages as well as be aware of its disadvantages. This is why you are likely only to be asked about a procedure that actually appears in your log book.

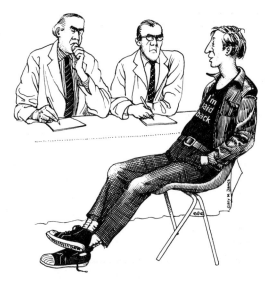

Fig. 16.1 Too casual an approach.

In spite of this, if it becomes apparent that the examiner does not accept or like your answer, do not persist in arguing — it is of significant negative benefit.

- Be too rigid. If the examiner wants you to discuss some other aspect of the subject, don't keep going regardless on your previous tack, as it will only annoy the examiner. Be adaptable to his or her wishes.
- Keep going after the bell. Many candidates have failed themselves by going on after the bell has sounded, and, in the heat of the moment and with relief that it is all over, have said something stupid with disastrous results.
- Give unrequested information — it can so easily provide a pitfall, or sidetrack the examiner into a field of discussion that is even more difficult and dangerous.
- Mention rarities first — always mention common things first.
- Sit there blankly if you are asked something that you don't know. If you don't know the answer or cannot work it out, then you must say so, and the examiner will change tack.
- Answer questions either by repeating them or by asking the examiner a question in reply. This is likely to evoke the response 'I am the one asking questions around here.'
- Give multiple treatment options if the examiner asks you how *you* would manage a specific condition or situation. He is

genuinely interested in how *you* would tackle that problem, not how everybody else may have approached it over the last decade.

- Be too hesitant — this suggests that you are *not* ready to take the examination.
- Take the examination too early — it can weaken morale if you fail badly.
- 'Waffle' and wave your hands around aimlessly. Try to make every word and movement count.
- Be irrational just because you are in an examination. Similarly don't skimp on your examination of a lesion — do it properly and in the right order. Remember your examination technique is as important as arriving at a correct diagnosis.
- Be too 'cocky' or overconfident. Aim for confident humility.
- Give up or lose your temper or calmness if you think you have failed in any section of the examination. You cannot be sure of the final outcome until the results are announced.

Finally...

Try to remember that the examiners are actually human (or reputedly so) and, whether you believe it or not, are actually doing their best to help you pass.

Whatever happens, try to display enthusiasm for the whole subject of *surgery* — it's a great career. If you don't succeed at first, try, try, *try* again.

The very best of luck!

Appendix 1
Approved
abbreviations

The following are approved abbreviations for use in the multiple-choice papers as published by the Royal College of Surgeons of England. This list is presented to each candidate within the 'Advice to candidates on the multiple choice question papers' and with each paper.

ACE	Angiotensin converting enzyme
ACTH	Adrenocorticotrophic hormone
ADH	Antidiuretic hormone
AIDS	Acquired immune deficiency syndrome
AIS	Abbreviated injury score
APACHE II	Acute physiological and chronic health evaluation II scoring system
APTT	Activated partial thromboplastin time
ARDS	Adult respiratory distress syndrome
ASA	American Society of Anaesthesiologists
BMI	Body mass index
BP	Blood pressure
BRCA1	Breast cancer gene 1
CAPD	Continuous ambulatory peritoneal dialysis
CDH	Congenital dislocation of the hip
CEPOD	Confidential enquiry into peri-operative deaths
CPAP	Continuous positive airway pressure
CSF	Cerebrospinal fluid
CT	Computed tomography
CVP	Central venous pressure
DTPA	Diethylene tetramene pentaacetic acid
DU	Duodenal ulcer

ECG	Electrocardiograph
EEG	Electroencephalograph
EMG	Electromyograph
ERCP	Endoscopic retrograde cholangiopancreatography
FEV_1	Forced expiratory volume in one second
FNA	Fine needle aspiration
FVC	Forced vital capacity
GCS	Glasgow coma scale
GI	Gastrointestinal
HCG	Human chorionic gonadotrophin
HDU	High dependency unit
HIV	Human immunodeficiency virus
IgA	Immunoglobulin A
IgD	Immunoglobulin D
IgE	Immunoglobulin E
IgG	Immunoglobulin G
IgM	Immunoglobulin M
INR	International normalized ratio
ISS	Injury severity score
ITU	Intensive therapy unit
IVC	Inferior vena cava
IVU	Intravenous urogram
JVP	Jugular venous pressure
LFTs	Liver function tests
MCV	Mean corpuscular volume
MEN	Multiple endocrine neoplasia
MESS	Mangled extremity severity score
MIBG	Meta iodo benzoyl guanidine
MMS	Mortality and morbidity score
MRI	Magnetic resonance imaging
PTFE	Polytetrafluoroethylene
PTH	Parathyroid hormone
QRS	Cardiographic wave form

RBC	Red blood cell
RTS	Revised trauma score
SIMV	Synchronized intermittent mandatory ventilation
SIRS	Systemic inflammatory response syndrome
SVC	Superior vena cava
TFTs	Thyroid function tests
TRISS	Trauma revised injury severity score
TSH	Thyroid stimulating hormone
VMA	Vanilylmandelic acid
WBC	White blood cell

Appendix 2
Glossary of conventional terms

Every effort is made in the setting of the multiple choice questions to ensure that the wording is as clear and unambiguous as possible. For further clarity and for the purpose of the MRCS examination the Royal College of Surgeons of England has published the following list of conventional terminology and their intended meanings. This list is presented to each candidate within the 'Advice to candidates on the multiple choice question papers' and with each paper.

Timing of surgery

Definitions are based on the Department of Health recommendations:

Immediate	Within 3 hours
Urgent	Within 24 hours.

Terminology

Characteristic, classical, predominantly and reliably:
> Imply that a feature would occur in at least 90% of cases.

Typically, frequently, commonly and usually:
> Imply that a feature would occur in at least 60% of cases.

Often and tends to:
> Imply that a feature would occur in at least 30% of cases.

Has been shown, associated, recognized, treatment of choice, optimally, adequately and features which may be present or may be caused by:
> Refer to evidence which can be found in a modern authoritative medical text. None of these terms makes any implication about the frequency with which the feature occurs.

Figures

When figures are given in the context of epidemiology, round figures are to be treated as approximations and precise figures as exact values:

For example, the figure of 30% does not imply exactly 30% but approximately 30% to within 5% either way. Conversely, the figure of 2% would mean precisely that amount is indicated.

Appendix 3
Recommended reading

Journals

British Journal of Surgery
Annals of the various Royal Colleges of Surgeons
British Medical Journal
British Journal of Hospital Medicine
Hospital Doctor
Hospital Update
Surgery (UK)

Distance learning

The STEP course (Royal College of Surgeons of England)

Anatomy

McMinn R M H 1994 *Last's anatomy*, 9th edn. Churchill Livingstone, Edinburgh

McMinn R M H, Pegington J, Abrahams P H 1993 *A colour atlas of human anatomy*, 3rd edn. Mosby, St Louis, USA

Physiology

Berne R M, Levy M N 1995 *Principles of physiology*. Mosby, St Louis, USA

Pathology

Kumar V, Cotran R S, Robbins S L 1997 *Basic pathology*, 6th edn. W B Saunders, Philadelphia
Walter J B, Israel M S 1996 *General pathology*. Churchill Livingstone, Edinburgh

Short textbooks

Burkitt H E, Quick C R G, Gatt D, Deacon P J 1995 *Essential surgery*, 2nd edn. Churchill Livingstone, Edinburgh

Dunn D C, Rawlinson N 1991 *Surgical diagnosis and management*. Blackwell Scientific, Oxford

Forrest A P M, Carter D C, Macleod I B (eds) 1995 *Principles and practice of surgery*, 3rd edn. Churchill Livingstone, Edinburgh

General textbooks

Burnand K G, Young A E (eds) 1998 *The new Aird's companion in surgical studies*, 2nd edn. Churchill Livingstone, Edinburgh

Kirk R M, Mansfield A O, Cochrane J (eds) 1996 *Clinical surgery in general*, 2nd edn. Churchill Livingstone, Edinburgh

Mann C V, Russell R C G, Williams N S 1995 Bailey and Love's *Short practice of surgery*, 22nd edn. Chapman & Hall, London

Emergency surgery

Ellis B 1995 Hamilton Bailey's *Emergency surgery*, 12th edn. Butterworth-Heinemann, Oxford

Physical signs

Browse N 1997 *An introduction to the symptoms and signs of surgical disease*. Edward Arnold, London

Others

Apley A G, Solomon L 1994 *A concise system of orthopaedics and fractures*. Butterworth-Heinemann, Oxford

Blandy J P 1998 *Lecture notes in urology*. Blackwell Scientific, Oxford

Hornick P, Lumley J, Grace P 1997 *Case presentations for the MRCS and AFRCS*. Butterworth-Heinemann, Oxford

Kirk R M 1994 *General surgical operations*, 3rd edn. Churchill Livingstone, Edinburgh

Recent advances in surgery (series). Churchill Livingstone, Edinburgh

Skinner D, Driscoll P, Earlam R 1996 *ABC of major trauma*, 2nd edn. BMJ Publications, London

Appendix 4
Normal values

It is important to realize that the values of the following will vary from laboratory to laboratory. However, it is advisable to have some idea of the normal range of values to be expected, and to quote them in SI units.

Blood

Haemoglobin	13–16 g/dl
Red blood cell count	4–$5 \times 10^{12}/l$
White blood cell count	4–$10 \times 10^{9}/l$
Platelets	150–$400 \times 10^{9}/l$
Packed cell volume	0.45
Prothrombin time	10–12 s
KCCT	26–38 s
Folate	2.5–15 µg/l
Vitamin B_{12}	140–590 pmol/l
pH	7.35–7.42
pO_2	10.5–13.5 kPa
pCO_2	4.5–6.0 kPa
Bicarbonate	20–30 mmol/l
Sodium	130–145 mmol/l
Potassium	3.5–5.0 mmol/l
Chloride	96–106 mmol/l
Urea	2.0–8.0 mmol/l
Creatinine	50–120 µmol/l
Uric acid	0.1–0.4 mmol/l
Calcium	2.02–2.66 mmol/l
Calcium adjusted	2.02–2.66 mmol/l
Phosphate	0.8–1.6 mmol/l
Total protein	65–80 g/l
Albumin	30–50 g/l

Globulin	20–35 g/l
Bilirubin	2–14 μmol/l
AST	10–35 U/l
ALT	10–30 U/l
GGT	5–50 U/l
Alkaline phosphatase	60–300 U/l

Urine

24-hour sodium	Up to 200 mmol
24-hour potassium	60–80 mmol
24-hour urea	410 mmol
24-hour protein	0.05 g
24-hour calcium	2.5–7.5 mmol
Creatinine clearance	1.2–2.3 ml/s
24-hour VMA	Less than 35 μmol
24-hour 5 HIAA	15–88 μmol

Appendix 5
Useful addresses

The Royal College of Surgeons of England
Examinations and Education Depts
35–43 Lincoln's Inn Fields
London WC2A 3PN
United Kingdom

The Royal College of Surgeons of Edinburgh
Nicolson Street
Edinburgh EH8 9DW
United Kingdom

The Royal College of Physicians and Surgeons of Glasgow
242 St Vincent's Street
Glasgow G2 5RJ
United Kingdom

The Royal College of Surgeons in Ireland
123 St Stephen's Green
Dublin 2
Republic of Ireland

Index